Make the Mind-Body Connection

In *Ayurvedic Balancing,* fitness professional Joyce Bueker shares what she learned on her journey to self-understanding.

First, you will get to know yourself. Learn about the three mind-body types, the three states of being, and the six tastes and their influence on lifestyle. Identify and explore imbalances, as well as hunger caused by over-grown appetites, dieting and deprivation, or emotional hunger.

Once you learn what's eating you, learn what to eat. A seven-day menu of recipes helps you adjust your palate to a more Ayurvedic, balanced, and sat-isfying way of eating.

You'll learn how to build a foundation for well-being through creative problem solving and tools for change. Identify and achieve healthful goals by envisioning abundant choices rather than focusing on deprivation or limita-tions. Reduce stress through meditation and guided imagery. Learn about exercises compatible with Ayurvedic balancing and ways of shifting your body's composition from fat-storing to fat-burning.

Finally, you'll learn to maintain balance through the naturally occurring flow of change within yourself as the seasons change. According to Bueker: "Creating abundance in life is like growing a very personal garden: you get to nurture your thoughts, emotions, and physical body, weeding out what does-n't work while observing the actions that help you to grow and thrive."

Bueker spent nine years lecturing and teaching workshops on weight management and maintaining a healthful lifestyle before being sidelined by an injury. Her quest for restored health led her to Yoga and Ayurvedic health practices. She now incorporates Ayurvedic principles into her work as a per-sonal fitness trainer, Yoga instructor, and lifestyle coach.

About the Author

Joyce Bueker (California) grew up in Texas where she graduated from the University of Texas in Austin with a B.A. in History. After spending time in Spain, attending the Institute of Language and Culture at the University of Navarre in Pamplona, she completed her Master's Degree in Modern Social History at Lancaster University in England. As an athlete, Joyce competed as an amateur competitive bodybuilder for nine years, culminating in the winning of her division in a U.S. national qualifying tournament (as seen on ESPN) and participation in national competition.

With eighteen years of experience in the fitness industry, including personal training and sports modeling as well as programming, sales, general management and marketing of health clubs, Joyce is also a second-degree Reiki practitioner, student of Okinawan Karate, Feng Shui, and Chinese Soaring Crane Qigong, and author of an autobiographical book of poetry titled *Seven Points of Light*. Joyce lives in the San Francisco Bay area. She loves the outdoors and enjoys hiking, biking, and caring for her family and ever-evolving garden.

To Write to the Author

If you wish to contact the author or would like more information about this book, please write to the author in care of Llewellyn Worldwide and we will forward your request. Both the author and publisher appreciate hearing from you and learning of your enjoyment of this book and how it has helped you. Llewellyn Worldwide cannot guarantee that every letter written to the author can be answered, but all will be forwarded. Please write to:

Joyce Bueker
℅ Llewellyn Worldwide
P.O. Box 64383, Dept. 0-7387-0188-2
St. Paul, MN 55164-0383, U.S.A.

Please enclose a self-addressed stamped envelope for reply, or $1.00 to cover costs.
If outside U.S.A., enclose international postal reply coupon.

Many of Llewellyn's authors have websites with additional information and resources. For more information, please visit our website at:

www.llewellyn.com

An Integration of Western Fitness
with Eastern Wellness

AYURVEDIC BALANCING

Joyce Bueker, M.A.

2002
Llewellyn Publications
St. Paul, Minnesota 55164-0383, U.S.A.

First Edition
First Printing, 2002

Book design and editing by Michael Maupin
Cover art © 2002 Lotus Flower Photodisc
Cover design by Lisa Novak
Interior illustrations by Mary Ann Zapalac
Poetry on part pages from *Seven Points of Light* by Joyce Bueker

The publishers have generously given permission to use extended quotations from the following copyrighted works. *Ayurvedic Cooking for Westerners* by Amadea Morningstar reprinted with permission from Lotus Press, Twin Lakes, Wisc., © 1995. All rights reserved. *Prakriti: Revised Enlarged Second Edition* by Dr. Richard Svoboda reprinted with permission from Lotus Press, Twin Lakes, Wisc., © 1998. All rights reserved. *Yoga & Ayurveda* by Dr. David Frawley reprinted with permission from Lotus Press, Twin Lakes: Wisc., © 1999. All rights reserved. *Ayurveda* by Vinod Verma used by permission from Samuel Weiser, York Beach: Maine. © 1995. *The New Life Library: Ayurveda* by Sally Morningstar first published by Lorenz Books, London, © 1999. *Perfect Health* by Deepak Chopra, copyright © 1990 by Deepak Chopra. Used by permission of Harmony Books, a division of Random House, Inc. *Ayurveda: A Life of Balance* by Maya Tiwari published by Healing Arts Press, an imprint of Inner Traditions International, Rochester, Vt., copyright © 1995 by Maya Tiwari. *The Book of Ayurveda* by Judith Morrison, adapted with permission of Simon & Schuster, copyright © 1995 by Gaia Books Ltd.

Library of Congress Cataloging-in-Publication Data
Bueker, Joyce, 1959–
    Ayurvedic Balancing : an integration of Western fitness with Eastern wellness /
    Joyce Bueker.
       p. cm.
    Includes index.
    ISBN 0-7387-0188-2
    1. Physical fitness—Psychological aspects. 2. Yoga. I. Title.
    GV481.2 .B84 2002
    613.7'046—dc21
    2001050442

Llewellyn Publications
A Division of Llewellyn Worldwide, Ltd.
P.O. Box 64383, Dept. 0-7387-0188-2
St. Paul, MN 55164-0383, U.S.A.
www.llewellyn.com

♻ Printed in the United States of America on recycled paper.

Many, many thanks
to Chris and Marcella for their love and support;
to Richard for his guidance; and
to Rob, whose own dedication to personal growth
helped me to "stay with it" and lay the foundation
for a most rewarding search.

Contents

List of Tables and Figures

Introduction

Most people over time develop a certain amount of skill to cope with life changes, stress, and personal growth. Modern Western culture has developed some specific responses to the challenges of our times: stress-management programs, self-help books, and the proliferation of health clubs, nutrition programs, and exercise fads. Often, stress- and time-management programs provide practical steps for individuals to feel more organized and relaxed, while the self-help movement has empowered many to develop a deeper awareness and understanding of nurturing their own physical, emotional, and mental well-being. And the great desire by Westerners to get in shape has led them to become proactive in their quest for physical wellness.

Western fitness—like its counterpart, Western medicine—is now stressing importance on preventative wellness and daily self-care, even though too often the focus is still on treating the immediate symptoms of discomfort and unhappiness without finding and treating the root of the problem. We procrastinate until weight problems, back pain, and stiffness become acute and bring us out of balance, and then crave instant gratification to ease our misery. Diets abound, with conflicting information and inconsistent results. More and more fitness enthusiasts are turning to Yoga and Ayurveda, because these Eastern approaches offer a more comprehensive definition and approach to wellness.

Yoga and its "sister science" Ayurveda (which has been around for thousands of years and literally translates as "life science") are Eastern philosophical and therapeutic responses to people's need to understand who they are, and create health on physical as well as mental and emotional levels. There is great benefit in studying Eastern and Western approaches to wellness, although it takes effort to assimilate both perspectives. For most busy Westerners, patience is an attribute not easily acquired, although more mindful practices such as Yoga postures, Ayurvedic nutrition, and meditation or quiet contemplation, build strength in this area over time. *Ayurvedic Balancing* serves as a starting point for Westerners to learn about basic principles of Ayurveda and Yoga in order to create a more well rounded and sustainable personal foundation for fitness and well-being in everyday life.

Like self-help, Ayurveda and Yoga ask us to become aware of problems, treat them, and then build a program for sustainable change. The goal is the same: to address the deeper dysfunction and create a truly personal approach to wellness that evolves with a person's changing needs. Often, however, cultural and spiritual (bordering on religious) overtones associated with the teaching of Yoga and Ayurveda become obstacles for learning, seemingly conflicting with Western values rather than complementing them. In addition, there are times when the fast pace of Western life makes us too impatient to slow down and acquire some of the skills that Eastern wellness practices offer, and there are times when these Eastern ways seem too esoteric and impractical for our modern perspective.

It is encouraging that, from a Western point of view, the pursuit of fitness is no longer a quest for the perfect body, but now encompasses programs for inner and outer health, to give a person an improved sense of well-being. So many times, however, people embark on fitness routines and diets only to get sidetracked by too many choices, too many demands from other aspects of their lives—leaving them with a sense that "something was missing" in their attempts to get in shape. When as individuals we realize that we may take responsibility for our health and define personal wellness in broader terms to include all aspects of well-being, then we begin to remove the stumbling blocks and built-in obstacles to attaining our fitness and wellness goals.

Ayurveda and Yoga offer us a comprehensive, thoughtful framework for the growth of mind, body, and spirit by focusing on the daily pursuit of physical, mental, and emotional health. Ayurvedic principles are general in nature and do not exclude a person's individual needs; in their broadest sense, Ayurvedic ideas are useful to understand how common characteristics that we all share manifest in ways that are unique to each individual. *Ayurvedic Balancing* applies these principles to a Western fitness environment and examines specific imbalances, which disrupt the achievement of our wellness goals. In our modern world, almost everyone has struggled at one time or another with stress reduction and weight management. All too often the sources of imbalance come from a lack of organized perspective and an unawareness of unmet "hungers"—whether literal, or metaphorical, or both—that manifest on physical, mental, and emotional levels.

For example, people who want to get in shape often begin by addressing their physical needs, such as the desire to lose fat, strengthen muscles, or increase flexibility. They make a commitment by joining a fitness facility and getting instruction, but often fail in their objectives because other aspects get in the way, or perhaps because their expectations of what their bodies and minds can do are too unrealistic. Factors such as self-motivation, natural tendencies of different types of physiques, emotional connections to self-image and food, and previous personal history all help or hinder the pursuit and achievement of a fitness goal. We look at ourselves subjectively—and perhaps unforgivingly—and so our conclusions about ourselves are usually too harsh or unrealistic or unclear. Ayurvedic principles give us a framework to better understand our imbalances in a more objective way so we may create positive, sustainable changes. *Ayurvedic Balancing* will help you apply these principles in a truly personal way, so that in your quest for fitness, who you are and what you want eventually coincide with what you really need.

There are many good books that describe and explain Ayurveda and Yoga, but to a Westerner interested in learning basic principles, often the ideas seem too overwhelming or unfamiliar to embrace. This book specifically discusses the typical obstacles encountered by Westerners trying to incorporate Eastern wellness into a Western fitness lifestyle. A few Ayurvedic books present a more Western approach to Ayurvedic nutrition, but do not fully address the need for Westerners to understand the emotional hunger of dieting or the importance of a healthy achievement drive. Nutritionally speaking, Ayurvedic books often focus on what a person shouldn't eat, which to a chronic dieter is an instant turn-off. In traditional Ayurvedic cooking, many of the ingredients are unfamiliar to Westerners, and so the principles of Ayurvedic nutrition, which may be acquired bit by bit over time, get shoved aside as too hard, too esoteric, too unpalatable for the Western lifestyle.

Ayurvedic self-care practices may also seem too foreign to people used to a Western environment, even though the principles behind the specific practices are universal in nature and applicable to people of differing physiques, cultures, and beliefs. In addition, Yoga is often viewed as a collection of exercises designed for people who are already limber, rather than as a therapeutic system to help people of any age and condition gain physical and mental flexibility. Also, the introspective or meditative aspect of many Eastern philosophies often get tangled in cultural or religious beliefs, or are seen as too ungrounded or even ridiculous. Enthusiastic instructors may often unknowingly imply that a person must become a part of a cultural, religious, or philosophical system to reap the benefits of an Ayurvedic or Yoga practice. Even though the teaching of Yoga and Ayurveda is still in its infancy in the West in terms of organization and consistency—echoing the growing pains of massage therapy, acupuncture, aerobic dance, and personal fitness training in recent years—there is much to be learned from a more Eastern approach to wellness. Ayurvedic Balancing discusses the obstacles of learning about Yoga and Ayurveda and offers a step-by-step approach to integrating specific Eastern wellness principles into a Western fitness lifestyle.

Using Ayurvedic principles may help a person create a perspective of abundance, by helping to satisfy unmet "hungers" on physical, mental, emotional, and even spiritual, levels. Using Western proactiveness from our knowledge of fitness, emotional growth, and goal achievement—and Eastern introspection and expanded notions of wellness—this book addresses the Western quest for more holistic weight and stress management. By integrating Ayurveda, Hatha Yoga, Western psychology, and fitness into sustainable habits, we may build and maintain a more balanced, sustainable foundation for personal wellness. It can be difficult to make significant lifestyle changes when most of us are overwhelmed by the basic "struggles" to eat enough veggies, get enough exercise, find enough leisure time, or stay motivated to achieve our fitness goals. Looking at Ayurvedic nutrition and Yoga postures from a literal as well as metaphorical perspective, *Ayurvedic Balancing* offers tangible ways to reduce "hunger" and gain a sense of equilibrium and perspective. The book also discusses the psychology behind fitness imbalances and offers tools for constructive, lasting change.

The quest for integrating physical health and sense of well-being into our daily lives can be an arduous but ultimately satisfying task. For Westerners, the fitness industry gives insight on exercise, nutrition, and self-motivation, and participating in self-help and stress-management programs may help us become aware of deeper needs and skills for coping with life's ups and downs. Studying Yoga and Ayurveda may also help us create a deeper understanding of what it means to feel in balance. Ayurvedic principles are broad enough to apply to all physical, mental, and emotional constitutions—they serve as a reference point to create a practical framework for wellness. More specifically, the application of Ayurveda occurs on an individual level, helping each person to observe his or her own creative and destructive tendencies, and use that information to ask the fundamental question: "What does it mean for me to be in balance?"

Ayurvedic Balancing is a step-by-step process of building a personalized foundation for wellness. So often it seems that making changes for the better are too overwhelming, too difficult, too inaccessible. Often we desire change but don't know where to begin. By introducing more balance into our busy modern lives, we may create a more comfortable lifestyle that supports healthy weight- and stress-management goals and personal growth in a clearer and less judgmental way. By discovering and accomplishing small, tangible steps, we may create a personalized approach to gaining and maintaining balance. The following are some possibilities.

Working with my unique mind-body combination I may learn to:

- Gain an understanding of my attributes and how they help shape who I am

- Discover the imbalances that affect my health and sense of well-being

- Understand these imbalances and why they manifest, so I may accept my current situation as an invitation to change

- Observe the link between "dis-ease" and my feelings of well-being, and the many kinds of hunger which are symptoms of imbalance

- Examine my resistance to change and feelings of deprivation, and expand my life choices

- Discover how to use my mind-body constitution to accommodate healthy changes in my self-image

As I create a lifestyle plan that works with my constitution I may:

- Understand my body composition and the lean-to-fat ratio

- Choose Ayurvedic-balancing foods that reduce hunger and stress

- Examine current eating patterns and their connections with past experience

- Become fed on all levels, working with emotional hunger and the instinctive body

- Harness my mind-body type to consciously increase my capacity for self-care

- Gradually shift my eating and living patterns as my habits of self-care expand

I may enhance my ability to manage personal growth as I:

- Use a goal-planning system to set positive, realistic goals

- Learn to use creative problem-solving skills to gain awareness of choices

- Create my own belief system that allows me to accept the rewards and setbacks of managing self-care

- Engage in physical activity to increase energy, strength, and flexibility (for body and mind) that agrees with my particular constitution and goals

- Allow time for meditation, study, and recreation or play, and nurturing to feed deeper need for peace and joy

- Learn to engage in fewer activities or goals in a given time, to enjoy the process of balancing

Ayurvedic Balancing: A Personal Perspective

The process of self-discovery can be a rather roundabout journey. In our inquiry, each of us resembles a young river meandering across a broad, flat, as yet featureless plain. Unconsciously and instinctively moving through what often seems unconnected incidences in our lives, we eventually gain a more conscious understanding of what it means to be individuals connected yet separate from other individuals. Over time we may grow into a greater understanding of who we are and what we wish to be through our wanderings and questionings as well as our confrontations and failures. Examining both painful and pleasant experiences helps us expand our self-awareness to a truly private level, making room for an internal view that includes our individual beliefs, not just those of the people and cultures that influence us.

The road to self-discovery allows us to create personal histories and perspectives from which we may look back and gather understanding as well as look forward to make choices about what we do and who we are. Just as a mature river deepens its channel and carves a more determined course through the surrounding terrain, we learn to make truly personal choices about our lives and our lifestyles, becoming more distinct in the process.

Studying history, specifically the physical, mental, and emotional patterns of people who have lived before us, gives us a starting point from which we may begin to unravel the mysteries of why we do what we do, and gain a sense of how we feel about it. When I was in college I had an instinctive sense that obtaining a degree in history would help me to know myself, even though humanistic studies have often been viewed as rather esoteric and of little importance in life. Nonetheless, I received my Master's Degree in Modern Social History from the University of Lancaster in England, where I focused on the impact of the Industrial Revolution on modern society. I found that making sense of contemporary history—that which is currently happening around us—was next to impossible, because as human beings we require a certain amount of perspective to be able to emotionally internalize the importance of these events as individuals, not just have an intellectual recollection of them. Looking at my own need to understand my actions and inclinations, I realize now why I was drawn to modern social history: I wanted to understand the impact of our high-tech, industrialized ways on my health, happiness, and sense of well-being.

I was in a lot of pain—physically, mentally, emotionally, and spiritually—and needed to make sense of the confusion I felt coming from my own family's version of dysfunction. I wanted to move on to a place of improved health and wellness. Acknowledging that just about everyone these days could consider themselves a "victim" or a "survivor" of a dysfunctional family, I needed to find ways to help myself feel well, productive, and in balance. I needed time to mature, to grow in comparative experiences and develop the capacity to feel and understand, and to work through my emotional responses about my past. Gaining an historical perspective of the world around me was important, even though it has taken me over twenty years understand some of what I was studying. It gave me the skill to become my own personal historian so I could gain objectivity and create a sustainable foundation for healthy living—a foundation that does not deny who I am but rather helps me focus on what I want to become by understanding my destructive tendencies and developing my creative ones.

Expanding my worldview to include studying the history of religion was the starting point in my efforts to create a more personal and inclusive view of spirituality. Choosing a career in fitness allowed me to expand my knowledge of health and self-care. And recovering from a bizarre neck injury in my thirties (believe it or not, I was hit in the back of the head with a waiter's tray at a restaurant!) eventually forced me to stop using work and athletics as distractions to my healing process. I turned to Yoga to regain strength and flexibility in my neck and back, and began to seek alternative health-care practices for immediate relief from my injury.

Eventually, I began to unravel the larger ball of yarn inside my head, and all my unanswered questions about my past poured out. Looking back at my earlier years, I had a lot of confusion to dismantle before I could choose lifestyle habits that truly nurtured my well-being. I was raised in an alcoholic home, where the emotional needs of my father overshadowed the needs of all others. In that environment, I did not learn how to cope with fear or pain but rather suppressed these feelings in an effort to "be strong," and the resulting need to overacheive and prove my self-worth manifested from my mid-teens through my early twenties as anorexia or self-imposed starvation, a striving for ultimate perfection which, as we all know, never comes. This overanxious state lead to nervousness about food, chronic digestive problems, and very low self-esteem. My ability to demonstrate accomplishment in athletics, academics, and career came (fortunately) from a big appetite for life and (unfortunately) from a strong need to control everything as a reaction to the upheavals of growing up in an emotionally insecure environment.

Through participation in self-help programs, courses on goal achievement, stress management, Eastern wellness practices, and a continued passion for fitness and nutrition, I began to find my equilibrium, and over time have acquired a better understanding of how to nurture myself and maintain a sustainable sense of well-being. I was particularly drawn to Yoga and

Ayurveda for their ability to give order and meaning to my meandering introspection. The study of these more Eastern viewpoints has, like the study of history, greatly complemented my own process of self-discovery. I have gained a perspective on wellness that has helped me create a personal framework from which I may fill in the missing (or connect together the rediscovered) pieces of understanding about myself. *Ayurvedic Balancing* is the result of my journey of self-discovery, and the desire to share these thoughts with fellow travelers. May it bring us peace.

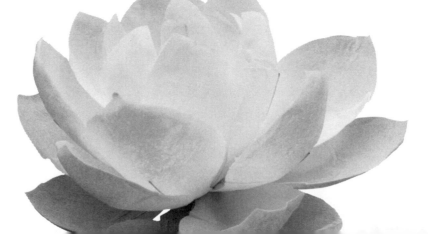

PART ONE

Defining Balance

This garden is not a place—
it's an awareness of all things growing:
seeds planted, flowers rising, fruits harvested,
and weeds to be pulled—
hunger and fullness
gathering and resting inside me . . .
My appetite for life having been restored
I am granted the hunger for balance.

1

ॐ

The Three Mind-Body Types

When trying to understand why we are the way we are, particularly in conjunction with an active desire to work with weight, stress, and personal growth issues, it is useful to have a definition of balance as a starting place for our inquiry. In the study of Ayurveda [i-yur-VAY-da], the sister science to Yoga whose literal translation means "life science," the definition of balance is universal in nature, containing common elements that are inclusive of all mind and body types; it is personal in nature, individualized to fit the unique attributes of each individual. This definition allows us to relate to characteristics everyone carries, as well as our own views of ourselves.

Often when we are under stress, or are continually displeased with our bodies, when we view ourselves as "less than on top of our game," we examine our less constructive tendencies too harshly. The concept of balance allows us to step back from our passions and see ourselves more objectively, and so more clearly see the thoughts and actions that combine to make up our distinct selves. As we learn more about the common tendencies within these mind-body types, we may then discover how these tendencies relate to our individual situations and conditions. Understanding our tendencies lets us examine those aspects of ourselves that keep us in balance and allows us less judgmental, more creative ways to view and address the causes of imbalance.

According to Ayurveda, everyone is made up of the same elements (ether, air, fire, water, and earth), and personal differences stem from the unique combinations of these elements in varying amounts as they manifest in physiological, mental, and emotional patterns. These elements combine to form three main mind-body types, or *doshas:*

Vata [VAH-tah]
- Airy and ethereal (manifesting as movement, breath, consciousness)

Pitta [PIT-tah]
- Fire and water (manifesting as metabolism, vitality, perception)

Kapha [KAH-fah]
- Water and earth (manifesting as bodily tissue, evenness, patience)

We all have these qualities in various and unique proportions, which make up our constitution or *Prakruti*, and usually two of the three types predominate, such as Vata/Pitta, Vata/Kapha, Pitta/Vata, Pitta/Kapha, Kapha/Vata, or Kapha/Pitta. In a balanced state, it is rare for a person to have a single predominating mind-body type or all three equally. However, a person can be in an aggravated condition and currently be overinfluenced by one category. In most cases, a person will have one mind-body type that will tend to be a predominate influence on physiology, thoughts, or emotions followed by a secondary type that, to a lesser degree, also manifests. The remaining mind-body type is also present but influences the person to an even lesser degree.

A good starting place for finding balance is recognizing and understanding both the nurturing and the disruptive qualities of your mind-body type, so you may increase and engage your positive, more constructive qualities to assist you in reaching your goals. Determining your mind-body type may be confusing at first, since sometimes you may identify with one grouping of characteristics, and at other times another. The more you begin to explore the combination of mind-body characteristics that creates your constitution, however, the more you will begin to learn which categories predominate and influence you most.

As you begin to identify characteristics specific to your constitution, you may also begin to notice similarities between yourself and life around you. In Ayurveda, not only are human aspects comprised of the five elements, but all aspects of life come from at least one of the five elements. It is helpful to look at these qualities from a broader perspective, and engage the imagination (and sense of humor!) while doing so. Looking at Ayurveda from a more metaphorical perspective will allow you to see a broader connection with life around you, while simultaneously gaining benefit from your introspection. In a mature Ayurvedic practice, a person can begin to feel in sync internally as well as externally with the surrounding environment. In this way, your sense of "feeling centered" has less likelihood of being disrupted by outside events; they are allowed in, but not blindly, maintaining your feelings of balance.

Table 1 (see page 6) describes the three main mind-body types in a worksheet format.* As you become more familiar with these terms and their qualities, you will begin to see how these attributes have shaped who you are, on physical, emotional, and mental levels. You may also gain insight into the constitutions and tendencies of those people around you. To determine your predominate mind-body category, put a checkmark in front of each line of characteristics (in each column) that best describes you when you are in a peaceful, healthy state, or perhaps the way you were as a child. Sometimes these characteristics may differ from your current condition, which is a clue to a potential source of irritation or imbalance.

If you are not sure if an aspect is your "true" nature but rather a response to an imbalance, indicate what is currently true for you. Count the checkmarks in each column, and add up your totals. The column with the greatest number of attributes marked is your primary mind-body type, and the column with the second greatest number of attributes marked is your secondary mind-body type, or dosha. As you become more familiar with your characteristics, your initial vision of your mind-body type may change, much like

* Table 1 includes information from various tables found in *Ayurveda, a Life of Balance* by Maya Tiwari (Healing Arts Press, Rochester, Vt., 1995).

	Ether/Air (Vata)	Fire/Water (Pitta)	Water/Earth (Kapha)
Skin	__ Dry, rough, cold __ Tan easily __ Premature wrinkling	__ Oily, soft, warm __ Tan moderately __ Freckles, moles	__ Cool, soft, dense, oily __ Pale, sunburns easily __ Smooth, fair
Hair	__ Brown or black __ Dry, thin, frizzy __ Tightly curled	__ Dark blonde, red __ Premature gray, bald __ Straight	__ Blonde, jet black, dk. brown __ Oily, abundant, shiny; __ Wavy
Eyes	__ Gray, brown or unusual __ Dull, narrow, small __ Dry, itchy	__ Lt. brown, hazel, green __ Almond shape, piercing __ Bloodshot, yellow sclera	__ Black, blue __ Big, bright, sensual __ White sclera
Frame and Face	__ Very short or tall __ Thin, big joints, flat chest __ Narrow face, bent nose	__ Medium build __ Athletic __ Angular face and nose	__ Heavy build __ Stocky, wide frame __ Round face, broad nose
Temperament/Thinking	*Imbalanced:* __ Nervous, indecisive __ Low tolerance to pain __ Fearful, frigid, blurred *Balanced:* __ Introspective __ Perceptive __ Disciplined, spiritual	*Imbalanced:* __ Arrogant, hot-headed __ Irritable, impatient __ Selfish, out-of-control *Balanced:* __ Alert, adaptable __ Intelligent, bright __ Successful	*Imbalanced:* __ Attached, greedy __ Stubborn, narrow- minded __ Neglectful, lazy *Balanced:* __ Calm, stable, forgiving __ Contemplative __ Nurturing
Food Consumption and Digestion	__ Like to snack __ Can be obese, addictive __ Constipation, gas	__ Good, yet irregular appetite __ Indigestion, ulcers __ Diarrhea, overspiced	__ Even appetite __ Over- or undereats __ Bloating, sluggishness
Total Attributes	_____	_____	_____

Table 1: The Mind-Body Types (Doshas)

layers of an onion peeled back to expose a core. It's all a part of the self-discovery process, which may be frustrating as you first begin to gather information, but rewarding as insight comes.

The Psychology of the Doshas

Now that you have begun to get an idea of your particular constitution, let's take a look at each dosha from a broader perspective.

Vata is a combination of ether and air. Consider the characteristics of ether and air: you know both exist but you can't actually see them, only their results. You can't see wind, but you see trees moving in the wind. Something that is ethereal does not exist literally, in a tangible, physical form, but rather in our minds and imaginations. Hence, Vata is a light, changeable, hard-to-pin-down quality; it's creativity and imagination, or playfulness and shyness. As represented in the seasons, Vata is found in the changeable seasons of spring and fall. Both seasons are transitions from definite states of hot and cold. Anyone who has ever tried to plant a vegetable garden can tell you that spring is unpredictable, with bursts of sunshine and warmth (should I plant those seeds now?), followed by dark clouds and rain (oops, the carrot seedlings just got washed away)—perhaps within moments of each other. Fall is a jittery time, too, with dry, brittle leaves carried capriciously by gusts of wind, with bursts of glowing, changing color against deep blue skies. Other examples in our world that illustrate the quality of Vata are quickly moving chipmunks always watchful for danger, or the fluffy foam on a cappuccino, or certain jobs such as a receptionist, whose job is juggling many tasks while conducting short, brief conversations with a variety of people.

In contrast to the lightness of Vata, Pitta is much more intense and purposeful. Composed of fire and water, Pitta is summer, the time of heat, thunderstorms, chili peppers, and an industrious time for growing crops. Pitta is athleticism, intelligence, the need to get things done and impatience when things aren't done correctly. Pitta is how you feel when someone cuts you off on the freeway in rush-hour traffic. Pitta can be very clear and to the point, and often offensive if the feelings of others are not taken into consideration. Pitta types usually take charge of a situation or exert leadership influences in some way. They are good at getting to the source of a problem. Pitta eyes see right through you, like a jackhammer rat-a-tat-tatting through to your bones. When Pitta is not balanced by rest and play, stress is the result.

Kapha, comprised of water and earth, has a much smoother quality than jumpy Vata or forceful Pitta. People with a lot of Kapha are usually well liked, as their natures tend to be more jovial and thoughtful of others. Kapha can be soothing, as a much deserved nap after a long hike, or numbing, as in watching too much TV and eating too many potato chips while on the couch. Steady movements, like a farmer plowing row after row after row with his tractor, are Kapha-like; so too is winter with its icy, wet weather, and animals who hoard food and hibernate through the cold. Kapha doesn't like letting go; they're like human pack rats, who collect lots of "neat stuff" (Pitta types, however, would refer to it as junk). It's hard to make Kapha people angry, but once you do, watch out—their long fuses have finally been lit, and a big explosion is likely to follow. Pittas quickly get mad and blow up, Vatas may hide anger in fear. Kapha has many sounds, like the soothing sound of waves coming onto a beach (or the sound of your partner snoring away in the middle of the night!).

Influences on Weight and Stress Management

Let's examine the mind-body types and their combinations from a weight and stress management perspective. Remember, none of the categories is more important or better than the others in terms of managing body fat, stress, or personal growth. In fact, each category has its strengths for moderating appetite and managing stress; conversely, each mind-body category has potential disruptive qualities, too, which are usually set in motion from an accumulation of insupportable habits, unawareness, natural changes, or possibly a life disruption of some kind.

Since Vata-type people are, on an essential level, influenced by the qualities of ether and air, they carry these same characteristics with regards to appetite and stress. In a healthy, relaxed state, Vata people are lighthearted and busy, often forgetting meals or leaving a sandwich half-eaten as they see or remember something else they want to do. It's ironic that Vata-influenced people often say they eat a lot, but when you actually watch them eat, they take forever to finish their food and many times don't even finish at all. They don't mind having a big meal and then waiting a long while for the next one, but heaven help the guy next to a hungry Vata person (crankiness is a clue here!). So if Vata appetites are irregular, and they get distracted by other things, Vata-influenced people in a healthy state don't think about food all that much and like expending energy. For weight management, less food combined with lots of activity usually means less physical weight.

What becomes difficult about this mind-body type with regards to weight management is when Vata is off-balance. If the less constructive aspects of Vata include nervousness, fear, and erratic appetite, then an imbalanced Vata can overeat when nervous, lonely, or emotional. Their appetites can be over-stimulated to make them hungry all the time, with the constant urge to nibble or munch. (And what in our modern world do we usually munch on but junk food, which satisfies the desire for stimulation of the sense of taste, but eventually makes us even hungrier!) Vata is the most sensitive of the three doshas; it is most easily thrown off balance because of its fragile nature. So Vata-influenced people who are under too much stress often use food as a buffer, a way to find immediate comfort. Food can be very comforting, especially in our age of abundance, with supermarkets filled with an incredible array of choices. As we shall see later, food eaten Ayurvedically can still be comforting—without being disruptive to weight, digestion, or energy levels.

Since predominantly Vata types have natures that tend toward nervous energy, a regular exercise pattern is beneficial for moderating this energy. So is a regular eating pattern, where appetite is tended to—like growing a well-tended garden, instead of allowing it to spill its plants in every direction. Specific habits with healthy intentions are greatly beneficial for Vata to feel balanced; the key is to not get stuck into old patterns that no longer serve. Fitness-oriented people who are primarily Vata types often become over-exercisers, relying on the frenetic expenditure of energy to balance weight instead of combining moderate exercise with quiet time (to soothe Vata's jumpiness) and regular food habits—which all combine to balance the appetite. However, the ability to be imaginative is also a Vata trait, so an inclination for a scattered approach to eating, exercising, and resting can also become a creative integration of personal time for nurturing, combined with a variety of recreational and exercise-oriented activities.

Vata people need variety. Diets seem too restrictive, and exercise becomes a burden when it feels forced or too rigid. People with a lot of Vata are usually small or thin-boned, and moderate training with weight equipment can be very beneficial for bone density and posture. However, if lifting weights is difficult or too intense, Vata people will often avoid this type of exercise (and the perceived discomfort that it brings) altogether, and therefore not receive its benefits. Workouts for Vata folks, therefore, need to be playful and varied, but with enough purpose to be effective.

Pitta influenced people, on the other hand, are much more likely to keep to an exercise routine because they like intense activity, and like the results even more. Bodybuilders and gymnasts remind us of muscularity and symmetry, both Pitta characteristics. Often, Pitta people love sports, and the "no pain, no gain" approach to exercise. Exercise may be used as a release from built-up pressures, since Pittas can accumulate during the day a lot of frustrated and sometimes angry feelings. Pittas mean well, but sometimes their insistence on perfection can lead to irritation with the rest of the world (which, unfortunately, isn't perfect), and the inability to quit a project or task to make room for regular rest and meals. If a Pitta person gets caught up in a task, the task takes priority over self-nurturing—which is why Pittas are often goal-oriented salespeople, project leaders, or CEOs who have a high potential for developing stress-related problems. Success, at any price, can be the motto of a Pitta not in balance with other needs.

Pittas who overwork often become overweight, since food becomes a way to soothe irritated nerves. A Pitta person normally has a well-developed appetite to begin with, and a powerful constitution, which can expend great amounts of energy. Too often, however, heated agitation from a fast-paced, intense day is too often placated by too many sweets and large meals. Combined with a tendency to sacrifice rest and exercise in order to accomplish a work goal, Pitta folks can often "eat their way" out of shape. Chapter 3 discusses in more detail the influence of the doshas on our sense of taste and the corresponding actions our "appetites" produce.

The quality of Pitta allows us to get motivated, focused, and disciplined enough to accomplish goals. Harnessing Pitta can be useful in engaging the intellect and becoming aware of the necessary influence of other doshas. If Pitta people can find a balance between work and play, they are capable of managing their weight and stress; first, however, they must learn to not be so hard on themselves (and others) as they invite balance into their lives.

Kapha influenced people, by their nature, are well equipped to maintain balance, as their temperaments tend to be even and calm. They also have great physical resiliency and show a much steadier pace for work and exercise. Like the proverbial tortoise and hare, Kapha people are steady and dependable tortoises, whereas Pitta people tend to burn themselves out if not mindful of their need for balance. Kapha people, therefore, have the ability to maintain a steady appetite and not "pig out" from exhaustion or nervousness. They seldom need breakfast and are happy with moderate meals. Their constitutions are strong, making them good for strength training and endurance events. They are not as distracted by the need to succeed or complete something (a Pitta trait) or the fear of failure (a Vata quality), so once they find a rhythm for work, rest, and play, Kaphas are able to navigate life's ups and downs well and maintain a sense of well-being inside.

If the quality of Kapha is brought out of balance, however, it can have damaging results to weight management and sustaining healthy habits. Kapha gives us a heightened appreciation of our senses, which often translates in our modern, overabundant world as a hunger for the finer things in life—good food, good drink, nice clothes, beautiful surroundings, and lots of time to spend enjoying these things. Kapha people are drawn to healthy, low-fat foods in a balanced state but heavier, calorie-rich foods when off-balance.

If the quality of Kapha, which by its nature desires calm and rest, gets understimulated, often only excess will do to placate a Kapha's need to overcome boredom. Probably all of us have all experienced the "couch potato" phenomenon, where physical, mental, or emotional fatigue leads us to overfeed our mouths and underfeed the need for release of pent-up feelings in healthy exercise or play. Kapha people are very tolerant, but this means that often they hold on to their feelings until their emotional reservoirs can't take anymore, and then they explode in anger or "numb out." As mentioned earlier, there is a direct correlation between the tastes we are drawn to and the actions we demonstrate, both in balanced and imbalanced states.

When Kapha is out of balance, weight gain is often a result. Kapha people tend to be heavier than other mind-body types, with bigger bones and more body tissue than Vatas and Pittas. Because our modern culture wrestles with the notion of thinness and self-esteem, Kaphas feel the most pressure to fit in to modern notions of what is attractive and desirable. Eating disorders and prolonged dieting are often experienced by modern-day Kaphas, and the subsequent frustration produced can turn the regularity of Kapha into sluggishness and apathy. Another aspect of Kapha is the tendency to feel understimulated, which in turn produces the need for excitement and adventure. The opposite is also true, namely, a Kapha person who is overloaded with work or feelings can simply shut down (figuratively, as in emotionally numb; mentally, as in unable to make a decision or implement a positive change; or physically, as in an underachieving couch potato). Kaphas are kept in balance when they are able to define clear goals and rewards for their efforts, and are given enough time and instances to satisfy their lust for life and need for play.

In summary, most people's constitutions give them constructive tendencies to feel balanced and well, as well as destructive tendencies that can bring undesired states of being. In addition, since we are comprised of all three mind-body categories to varying degrees, we may sometimes feel at odds with our own natures (a Vata/Kapha's need to be both active and relaxed). As we will see in chapter 2, often our balance is defined as a careful dance between the three states of being.

ॐ

The Three
Mind-Body
Types

2

ॐ

The Three States of Being

The desire to create and maintain a sustainable feeling of well-being or balance is a natural function of our constitutions; also existing is the tendency to disregard the signals that our mind-body types or doshas send us when an imbalance is occurring. Imbalances occurring in our doshas affect our state of being. The three states of being are:

Sattvic
- Equilibrium, healthy curiosity, and the ability to think

Rajasic
- Motion, the urge to reorganize or manifest

Tamasic
- Inertia, a desire to stop and rest

Food may be described by these states: *sattvic* (balancing), *rajasic* (heating or agitating), or *tamasic* (making cold or numb). A fresh peach on a warm summer day could be considered sattvic or balancing, as it appeases hunger and the desire for something tasty without creating heaviness or heating us up. A hot chili pepper is rajasic, as it stirs the metabolism and agitates the digestive juices. In contrast, a bowl of ice cream is heavy, filling, cooling to the mouth, and numbing to the digestion. As we will see in chapter 3, the achievement of a sattvic or balanced diet involves the physical sensation of taste; but it also involves our mental and emotional states. For example, enjoying the preparation and consumption of a healthy meal could be considered nurturing or sattvic. How we prepare our food, how we feel about eating in general and how we are feeling as we eat a specific meal all represent different aspects of creating a nurturing, balancing diet.

Thus not only the food we eat but the activities we engage in also have these qualities and affect our state of being. Taking a walk in a beautiful park nurtures the senses, calms the mind, and gives the body balanced exercise. Writing a term paper often stirs up thoughts, manifests ideas, and may be considered agitating or rajasic. Watching a movie while lying on the couch is inertia or a tamasic state. Our thoughts can be in a state of relaxation or meditation; they can be angry or indifferent, too. These three states of being describe our physical, mental and emotional states, and as we go through life we move from one state of being to another. Just as in nature, where we may see a certain logic and state of purpose to the transition of molten lava (rajasic) to a solid piece of rock (tamasic), our lives may flow from various states in a natural cycle—one that does not stop change, but that allows change to feel acceptable and okay.

Ayurveda is a study of the dance of the three states of being and how they affect our mind-body characteristics. Recalling the descriptions of the various doshas in chapter 1, the quality of Vata is one of movement. If the movement is agitated, as in a gust of wind, the movement is rajasic. If the movement is playful and appealing, as in a person "moving" his or her thoughts through a pleasant imagining (like a fun daydream or a creative moment when ideas are "flowing"), the state of being is nurturing or sattvic in nature. The quality of Pitta, by its very nature, is a quality of movement—of getting things done, of completing a task, of manifesting. If a person has a lot of Pitta in his or her constitution, the tendency for that person is to keep moving from activity to activity with intensity. There are different levels of exertion, and if the person is exerting effort but is in a relaxed state, the productivity is still present but the agitation level is lower. Therefore, Pitta people who do not develop other aspects of their constitution (which bring balancing rest and playfulness) often find themselves in an overintense or prolonged state of agitation, which may manifest as a tendency toward anger, overgrown appetite, burnout from stress, or even certain physical discomforts or illnesses. On the other hand, Kapha-influenced people may be the opposite, tending toward not enough movement in their mental, emotional, and physical states. A person "weighed down" by a Kapha imbalance has a hard time making a change or letting go of things and may manifest excess body tissue from lack of physical movement and making heavier, rather than lighter, food choices.

Just as our mind-body types offer us constructive tools to manage weight and stress (as well as potential tendencies for less constructive habits), our doshas are forever dancing between the different states of equilibrium, agitation, and inertia. To gain skill in consciously nurturing your state of mind, therefore, the study of Ayurveda asks you to become aware of your mind-body characteristics and the inherent tendencies and influences of those qualities on your state of being.

As a young child, most often a person is in a state of balance, moving from activity to rest in an unconscious but natural way. As we get older, we begin to become conscious of the ups and downs of life and get exposed to potentially imbalancing experiences which affect our states of mind and being. The growing pains of becoming a teenager; the challenge of earning a living and identifying a life course; being in relationship with family, friends, coworkers, acquaintances, and even enemies; experiencing traumas and joys and mysteries—all aspects of our lives are shaped and influenced by the dance of our doshas and how well we come to understand our inherent constitutions and needs.

For everyday purposes, the objective of balancing is not to hold onto a perfect state of equilibrium, because in a world of change and possibilities, that kind of perfection is not a probability. However, as we come to understand our natures and the kinds of actions which tend to bring us out of balance, we may choose to become more conscious of our constructive tendencies, and develop habits which begin to bring us into more moments of equilibrium that connect themselves over time into a feeling and sustainable state of well-being.

In Yoga, the objective of doing physical postures or *asanas* is not to achieve perfection but rather to move in and out of the pose with a relaxed but conscious purpose. If a person is physically challenged to accomplish a certain pose and finds himself or herself struggling to gain more strength, more flexibility or more breath, that person is attempting the pose in an increased state of agitation, which adversely affects his or her physical, mental, and emotional state. In Yoga class, both the new and the experienced student fall out of poses all the time; the difference between the two students is their states of being. Clearly, both are harnessing the energy of *rajas* or movement to accomplish the pose, but the more advanced student will go in and out of the pose with continued, expansive breathing (rather than groans, grunts and shallow gulps of air;) with an intellect that is more interested in focusing on the various physical cues to increase the sustainance of the pose (rather than becoming angry or frustrated when encountering limitations in one's flexibility, strength or ability to balance); and less emotional attachment to the outcome of the pose (rather than holding onto the "successful" or "unsuccessful" performance of the pose, or the emotions that the difficulty or pain or perhaps joy of the pose brought).

Over time, a Yoga student may become conscious of his or her thoughts, feelings, and actions in class to the point where the new state of consciousness becomes comfortable and natural. This more balanced approach to class allows the student to move into an unconsciously balanced state, where the student naturally seeks to perform the poses in a constructive way because the state of being produced is agreeable and nurturing (i.e., sattvic). If the student has good instruction and practices Yoga regularly, in time his or her approach to Yoga class spills over into all aspects of life, because in a healthy state, our doshas seek to integrate their qualities into a useful, nurturing state. In other words, our bodies, minds, and emotions naturally seek balance, if we develop habits which allow their healthy voices to be heard.

Let's examine two specific Hatha Yoga postures for their analogies to the concept of creating and maintaining balance or well-being. A standing balancing pose called the "Pulling Bow" requires great determination to keep balanced on one leg while moving the other leg and extended arm in opposite directions (see the figures on the following page). For a more advanced student, the extened leg is in one line with the standing leg; it took me a while before I could open up my tight hip muscles enough to extend my leg over my head at all. For me, the beauty of this pose is its symbolism of the dance of the doshas, the tug and pull of life and character traits which potentially pull us in all directions but can, like in this pose, be directed to achieve greater flexibility, grace and endurance of mind, body and spirit. As the extended leg is pushed upward, the extended arm reaches away from the leg. In other words, your mind is instructing your body to move in two opposite directions, and what allows you to move further in the pose is the ability to use the pulling arm to balance the opposing movements of pushing up and reaching out. This pose asks the student to become comfortable with the contradictions inherent in the pose and work with these opposing forces to balance each other, just as Ayurvedic Balancing asks us to recognize our conflicting tendencies and develop a consciousness about them, so we can "pull" ourselves this way or "push" ourselves that way when needed. Seeking and maintaining balance is an active state, one that always needs attention to maintain. Like the pose, the minute the leg pushes too hard, the balance between the tension is lost, and the student loses balance, eventually falling out of the pose. The student has the option, however, of trying the pose again, and over time building strength and awareness to grow in the pose (and so in its benefits). Over time, the movements become more subtle, and so more lasting and sustainable.

The second pose is aptly called "Balancing Stick." The foundation of the pose is created by first focusing on the source of strength: the standing leg, with foot firmly planted and the muscles in the front of the leg contracting

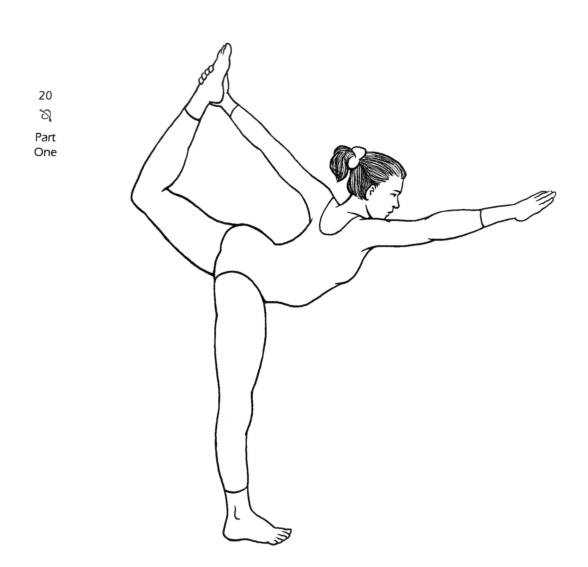

Figure 1: **The Pulling Bow**

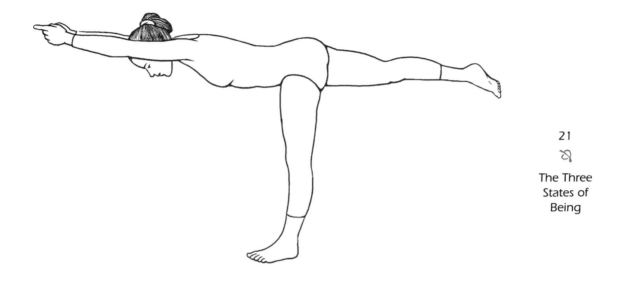

Figure 2: **The Balancing Stick**

tightly, pulling up from the kneecap. If a person could only stand upright on one leg and keep the focus on contracting the quadriceps muscles tightly (without even being concerned about extending the other leg and upper torso out, as the picture illustrates), that person would have accomplished a fundamental principle of creating a firm foundation before trying to accomplish a more advanced state. As my physical strength and focus of mind increases, the ability to go deeper into the pose develops. The strength of the standing leg contributes to the contraction of the abdominal muscles, which in turn allows me to hold my other leg and arms out. I have experienced moments when it felt like my arms and suspended leg were almost floating effortlessly, because I focused not on the difficulty of the pose, but on the steps necessary to perform it, which allowed me to engage my lungs, expand my ability to process oxygen, and therefore give me the endurance to sustain "Balancing Stick" pose (which is appropriately described by some as the marriage of heart and lungs). Even with heart pumping furiously and lungs expanding to get the most oxygen available, I was able to hold this pose, because my single-minded focus was to keep the foundation strong and keep pulling the muscles up around my knee-cap (while keeping the back of the knee somewhat loose, to avoid locking the knee and creating injury).

The dance of the doshas is evident here, as I kept my mind (and therefore arms and leg) light by focusing on performing certain physical tasks (engaging the leg muscles, abdominals, and lungs) rather than becoming worried that I wouldn't be able to fully achieve this "marriage between heart and lungs." I focused on what I could do, and so, in this case, performed the pose to a more advanced degree. Years ago I suffered a prolonged illness and injured my back, and could not do this pose at all. As I slowly started to recover, I experienced the frustration of knowing what I used to be able to do, contrasted with the reality of not being able to do the pose at all (except stand on one leg and work again to build a foundation of basic strength). But I also remembered the feeling of effortlessness I had once experienced, and so endeavored to do whatever part of the pose I could while maintaining a relaxed attitude.

This mental ability, to not worry about the outcome of the pose but rather put all my energy into the consistant, day-by-day practice of the pose, is much like a principle foundation of Ayurvedic Balancing: to concentrate energy on the constructive characteristics and traits and build them up over time. By focusing single-mindedly on what I could do, I was able over time to regain my strength, flexibility, and endurance. I've even been able to again feel the joy of effortlessness while performing Balancing Stick in a state of relaxed intensity, because I went back to the basics and put in the time and effort needed to re-create the foundation for strength, bit by bit, in my weakened leg. My goal was to put the skills learned in all the times I had previously performed Balancing Stick to good use by harnessing a relaxed state of mind and ability to focusing on physical cues to begin to gain strength in my legs, abdominal muscles, and lower back. The result: by not emotionally focusing on the outcome of my performance but by being willing to try again and again, I was able to maintain a sense of well-being. Performing the pose fully again was icing on the cake.

Yoga harnesses the mind to concentrate, to hear the body's subtle and not-so-subtle cues, to gain flexibility and strength in body and in thoughts. Yoga expands our ability to breathe to take in more oxygen for sustainance; Ayurveda allows us to create nurturing habits which keep our states of being more easily in balance. As one Yoga instructor once told me, don't worry about trying to learn how to breathe. Just release what is no longer needed (stale air) as much as you can, and the lungs will know what to do. If you open a space for exploration and expansion by identifying unproductive habits and learning new skills for self-nurturing, the constructive aspects of your doshas will tell you what to do. Learning how our sense of taste affects our food consumption and state of being is the next step in understanding balance.

3

ॐ

The Six Tastes and Their Influence

In *Ayurvedic* nutrition, there are six tastes that correspond to different elements and senses (see Table 2, following page).

Tastes not only affect our appetite and satisfaction from eating food; use (or overuse) of tastes affects emotions and mental states as well. According to *Prakriti* by Robert Svoboda:

> All Tastes can be used as intoxicants. Sweet, for example, is a popular drug in our society. People use it to make themselves feel satisfied. Some societies intoxicate themselves with the envy of Sour or the irritability of Pungent, and some individuals may even use Bitter and Astringent for self-gratification. We all use our food to alter our consciousness, and all alterations of consciousness affect the body via the Three Doshas [the three mind/body types] . . . .[2]

As we examine the influence of tastes, we see that "sweet" is often used in our society to reduce stress and placate hurts (remember the cookies we got after we scraped our knees as kids? Or the sweetness of a loved one picking us up and holding us until we stopped crying?). In our increasingly stressful, adult lives, we probably don't get enough "sweetness" to comfort the stresses of satisfying the expectations of others and of ourselves. Instead, we move in high gear all day long, and then collapse into evening, with food

	Composed Of	Influences
Bitter	Ether and Air	Vata, Hearing
Astringent	Air and Earth	Vata and Kapha, Touch and Smell
Pungent	Air and Fire	Vata and Pitta, Touch and Sight
Sour	Fire and Earth	Pitta and Kapha, Sight and Smell
Salty	Fire and Water	Pitta and Kapha, Sight and Taste
Sweet	Water and Earth	Pitta and Kapha, Taste and Smell

Table 2: **The Six Tastes**

as a great and predominant placator. We can begin to see how compelling it is to consume large quantities of fat, refined sugar, and salt as they numb us, quell us, and overstimulate our senses. A major problem with this cycle, as it relates to our ability to really taste our food and enjoy our lives, is that our tastebuds and sensory abilities get overloaded. We become numb to the subtleties of the tastes in food as well as numb to the fatigue of doing too much everyday, or doing things which habitually do not feed us on our deeper levels, and thus we use food and distractions to cover up deeper imbalances. What we "taste"—in our food as well as in our lifestyles—does affect our physiology. Our emotions and mental patterns are also affected, further influencing the shape and wellness of our physical bodies.

A person may not rely on food to numb or stimulate the senses, but may do so emotionally or mentally, subconsciously choosing to avoid situations that seem too uncomfortable. Very often, people who are overweight (thus indicating a Kapha imbalance through an excess of tissue) are also out of balance in more fundamental ways. For example, a person who has a lot of intensity and is "driven" to achieve is manifesting a lot of Pitta, which is a heating property that may increase appetite for food and success to intense levels. Sometimes the symptoms of excess Pitta manifest as frequent expressions of crankiness or anger and criticism directed at the self or others. Often people running on excess "Pitta power" are not easily satisfied, doing way too much during the day and running themselves down into physical, emotional, and mental exhaustion. When the end of the day comes, food choices overwhelmingly shift to sugar, fat, and salt because they immediate satisfy taste—unfortunately with unwanted side effects. The body's unchecked appetite is a symptom of an unchecked lifestyle which is not "getting fed" all of what it needs, including clearer thoughts and necessary pauses in the hustle and bustle of achievement—which means that often a physical Kapha imbalance is symptomatic of a Pitta imbalance!

Underneath the drive to overperform may be another imbalance in the Vata quality, marked by a deep-seated lack of self-esteem or some message from the past, which unconsciously says that no matter what is done, it isn't good enough. Often these messages come from early traumas such as growing up in a dysfunctional home or being unmercifully teased or chided as a child for being too fat, too slow, too shy, too unattractive, etc. The deepest hunger of all is the unmet cry of a part inside that needs to be soothed. This imbalance in our more tender Vata quality creates a fearful response to life, and often that fear is shielded by a stimulation of the Pitta quality that allows us to survive, solve problems, and manifest our thoughts into meaningful action. Some Pitta is good, because it stimulates us to accomplish goals. If unchecked, however, excess Pitta can lead us beyond meaningful accomplishments into the world of excess "busy-ness" and accomplishment as a way to ignore deeper feelings of anxiety or insecurity. In other words, some Pitta helps balance the fearful tendencies of Vata; if those fears are deep-seated and not eventually addressed, an imbalance of too much Pitta may occur, and our achievement drive is stuck on overdrive (a condition which often leads to yet another imbalance—an increase in Kapha to "cool down" the excess of overheated Pitta).

Another Vata imbalance that leads to undesirable weight gain is caused by a lack of the Pitta quality to focus and organize, which leaves excess Vata confused and unfocused and eventually manifests as erratic, nervous, or compulsive eating habits. In weight management, being busy is not the same as having regular exercise, which brings the heart rate to a moderately and consistently raised elevation to assist the body in metabolizing fat. Often the fear of weight gain will increase an urge to always be busy (and therefore be burning calories); over time this increases the Vata quality to an imbalance and supercedes a more organized, thoughtful, and less emotional or fearful approach to weight management.

Thus an overintense, Pitta-type person or a nervous Vata person may learn to soothe high levels of overstimulation or stress with food, often resulting in the manifestation of excess tissues (a Kapha imbalance); while underneath the busy-ness, these people may really be feeding the unsoothed Vata imbalance which is broadcasting a silent but pervasive signal of emotional hunger. No matter how much "Pitta power" is solicited to bring discipline to a diet or exercise program, that underlying signal will do its best to undermine determination. The Vata imbalance is not there to keep this person eternally frustrated; it is there to allow him or her to come to grips with that which did not go well long ago.

Once the emotional pain is identified, it is easier to see the habits taken up over time which have progressively led to further imbalances: an insecurity, covered up/soothed/fortified by accomplishment that often manifests as compulsion for overstimulation and overaccomplishment, which often leads to an inflamed appetite, undesirable weight gain, and perhaps other health issues. Food is one of the most important aspects of our living. We plan our days around the preparation and/or consumption of it, we have special memories and emotional responses associated with it (the smell of a holiday dinner being a common image associated with good times and well-being), and so very often we create adversarial relationships with food because of the inability to understand and manage overgrown appetites and underfed senses of well-being.

Sometimes we use distractions such as busy schedules to ignore our needs for freshly prepared food. If our relationship with food may gradually shift back into healthier, more natural, and nurturing responses to the sensation of hunger, then our lifestyles shift, too. We begin to feed ourselves more of the "sweet" and healthy actions in life: laughter, playtime, less demands for perfection and more conscious achievement, and food that returns to us a more sensitive palate, bringing with it the joys and satisfaction of well-prepared, satisfying, and balancing meals. Numbness is a state of overload, when too many emotions and demands have been placed upon us. Gradually, with persistence and the desire for balance (after feeling the uncomfortable impact of imbalances,) we may shift into a more relaxed pace of meaningful activity, where nervous energy is soothed by rest, and the need to achieve is softened by the desire to enjoy the process of obtaining a goal and its rewards rather than being fueled strictly by the intense need to "get there."

We all have our tendencies, depending upon the combination of mind-body types which form our constitutions. Those with a lot of Vata energy require outlets for creative play and movement as well as regular habits and the understanding of fear which leads to courage without crushing sensitivity. Pitta folks may learn to harness their intellect and focus to create a softer lifestyle, using their intensity as an invitation for regular self-care and their intellect to develop a deeper understanding of the need for tolerance of others. Those with lots of Kapha begin to channel their gusto for sensory stimulation into a balanced routine of exercise, flavorful but lighter eating, and appreciation for rewards that come from focus, good choices, and patience over time.

Taste may then be harnessed to bring about balance, in body composition as well as lifestyle, and internal thoughts and feelings. A little bitter is good to

	Balanced By	Irritated By (Excess of)
Vata	*Sweet* (Heavy, moist, cool) *Sour* (Warm, moist, heavy) *Salty* (Heavy, moist, warm)	Pungent, bitter, astringent
Pitta	*Sweet* (Heavy, moist, cool) *Bitter* (Cold, light, dry) *Astringent* (Cool, light, dry)	Sour, salty, pungent
Kapha	*Pungent* (Hot, light, dry) *Bitter* (Cold, light, dry) *Astringent* (Cool, light, dry)	Sweet, sour, salty

Table 3: Effects of the Tastes on the Doshas

let us face reality—too much dries up our trust. Likewise, an astringent experience that helps us come to grips with loneliness and solitude helps us heal and regain our trust through introspection and self-nurturing. The rub is to then move past the dryness and drink in interaction again. Pungent activities are softened by an increased awareness of what obsession and sharpness do to ourselves and to others—perhaps goals may then become more like requests. A more grounded, saltier life with an understanding of the usefulness of moderation lets us taste life fully without the excess which causes undesirable imbalance. And we are balanced by the remembrance of bitter pills finally swallowed, sour memories finally acknowledged and released. Sweetness is again tasted and savored in more simple forms—literally we begin to taste the sweet stuff of our actions. Correspondingly, when the flavors of food begin to come back to numbed palates, the body's appetite is more easily satisfied. As we will see in Part 4, herbs, spices, and food choices that nourish our unique combination of mind-body attributes nourish our senses, too, without adding excess weight. We are invited to learn the fundamentals of taking care of ourselves through the nurturing practice of cooking nurturing food. With a few new habits, and time, balance becomes a known feeling again, and more often than not a regular state of being.

Table 3 on page 30 shows a summary of the effects of tastes on the three mind-body types.

The foods we eat, whether it be a vegetable or piece of fruit, grains or legumes, a spice or herb, meat or dairy, etc., is comprised of one or more of these six tastes. Since each mind-body type is enhanced or aggravated by certain tastes, it makes sense that the food choices we make affect us because they directly affect our individual mind-body types. For example, a person who has a lot of Vata in his or her constitution has a tendency to have dry skin and dryness of the digestive tract (as illustrated in Table 1, chapter 1,) so eating a lot of dry, snacky food would tend to increase the Vata to aggravated levels and create an imbalance as perhaps indicated by itchy skin, constipation, gas, or bloating. A person who by nature is rather intense and prone to anger (Pitta) is calmed by cooling foods such as dairy, but irritated by foods that have a lot of pungent ingredients such as onions, hot peppers, and garlic. Kapha by nature is cool and oily, so someone with a lot of Kapha in his or her constitution is well served by lighter foods such as salads with a moderate amount of fresh dressing rather than heavier foods made with excess oil.

4

Examining Lifestyle Imbalances

According to Ayurveda, our constitutions may be thrown off balance by influences such as physical environment, relationships, seasons, life changes, and temperaments. Judith Morrison, in *The Book of Ayurveda: a Holistic Approach to Health and Longevity*, discusses causes of imbalance and and how these imbalances affect our physical bodies, which is summarized in Table 4, following page.

Maintaining balance requires us to become aware of our external world as well as create an internal view of what balance means to us personally. As we begin to understand what keeps us in balance on all our levels of being— in our physical bodies, in our thoughts and actions, in our hearts and feelings, and in our spiritedness or essence—we begin to see those interactions that have caused imbalance. We begin to understand how an increase in one aspect of our constitution or makeup may increase that quality to an aggravated level, which may make us intolerant to even small amounts of something with qualities similar to that aggravated condition. We may also see how one aggravated aspect of our constitution may throw other aspects of our constitution out of balance as well.

Illness, excess weight and lethargy, emotional pain, and stress are all symptoms of deeper, more subtle imbalances trying to be expressed. Once uncovered, they find their voices in our thoughts and bodies and cry out to be heard, understood, tended to, and then released. In this way, the messages

Vata	Pitta	Kapha
Exposure to cold; fall/early winter	Exposure to heat; summer	Exposure to cold; late winter, spring
No daily routine	Perfectionist	Lack of motivation
Dry, frozen foods; leftovers; too much bitter, pungent, or astringent tastes	Red meat, salt, spicy, or sour foods; stressful (pungent) lifestyle that inflames appetite	Sweets, meat, fats, dairy and ice cream, fried foods, excessive salt
Missing meals, fasting	Indigestion, rushed	Eating w/o satisfaction
Too much travelling	Aggressive work	Underachievement
Too much or inappropriate exercise	Exercising at midday; competitiveness	Lack of exercise or movement
Misusing senses	Overthinking	Underuse of the senses
Alcohol, stimulants	Alcohol, antibiotics	Sedatives & tranquilizers
Too much sex	Lack of laughter, play	Oversleeping, naps
Not oiling dry skin	Excessive heat/sun	Excessive water intake
Too little sleep; working late nights	Fatigue, not knowing when to stop	Passiveness, boredom, coldness, indifference
Suppressing natural urges; abdominal surgery; colonics; suppression of anxiety, grief, fear	Anger, hate, fear of failure, and repression of these emotions	Doubts, greed, and possessiveness; staying attached to these emotions

Table 4: Imbalances and Their Causes

Vata	Pitta	Kapha
Influences:	*Influences:*	*Influences:*
brain, heart, colon, bones, lungs, bladder, nervous system	skin, eyes, liver, brain, blood, spleen, small intestine, endocrine	brain, joints, mouth, lymph, stomach, heart and lung cavities
Associated conditions:	*Associated conditions:*	*Associated conditions:*
backache, constipation, depression, sciatica, varicose veins, wrinkles	peptic ulcer, migraines, hypertension, colitis, weak liver, hemmorroids	bronchitis, emphysema, sinus congestion, headache, diabetes, sore throat, some forms of asthma

Table 4: Imbalances and Their Causes (continued)

of imbalance bring us the opportunity to regain balance, granting us the motivation to more readily embrace those daily aspects and habits that truly bring us life. At the same time we learn to accept our current conditions in a more kindly way while releasing what no longer serves our growth. We learn to let go of toxins that our overstimulated, modern lives have created and reduce the creation of new toxins by developing daily habits of awareness and self-care.

Introducing balance becomes a daily practice that feeds us and sustains us and satisfies us on all levels. Maintaining balance becomes more desirable and pleasurable rather than an overwhelming chore. As our lives manifest more moments of sweetness, less anger and sluggishness, our bodies consume less fats, sugars, and salts. And our minds and spirits begin to understand and embrace personal definitions of peace that nurture rather than numb our senses, without destroying the delicate interactions we have with others and with the environment. As we become aware of imbalance in our daily lives, we may learn to introduce small, careful, and individually agreeable changes that feed us on all levels. These new habits become the foundation for our self-care and sense of well-being and balance.

Discovering our imbalances can be an empowering, relieving, and restorative process when our intention is to incorporate balance on all levels. Merely treating symptoms will not satisfy our deeper needs; for example, dieting to lose fat without addressing the patterns and beliefs that brought us to dissatisfaction with our bodies may bring temporary weight loss followed by weight gain and an even greater sense of frustration and dissatisfaction. With some detective work and patience, we may apply Ayurvedic principles to our examination of these deeper needs, while addressing our more immediate desire for relief and tangible change. Before we create specific goals for change, however, we would be wise to examine on a broader scale those aspects which are causing imbalance.

Which current aspects negatively affect your physical, mental, or emotional well-being?

Life Aspect: Effect on Well-being:

Occupation:

Activities:

Relationships:

Physical environment:

Emotional environment:

Belief systems, attitudes:

Life Aspect:

Effect on Well-being:

Illness/impairment/trauma:

Food Consumption:

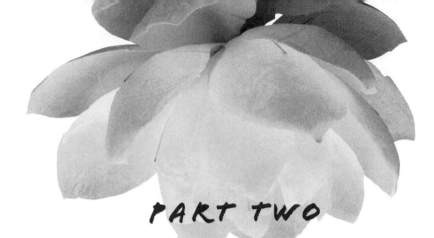

PART TWO

Indentifying
Hunger

*This is a journey that goes deeply
into the scared, scarred place
of my hunger and well-being*

*for all the work I've done
to get strong and whole and healthy
this place must be found
and transformed*

*it holds my happiness
it holds the tightness in me
and so my peace . . .*

5

Overgrown Appetites

In chapter 3, we discussed the connection between what we eat and how we feel, and how we feel and what we think and do. Since the West is a society with potentially overabundant choices, our culture often tends to be defined by extremes and excess rather than moderation and conscious decisions about how we live. As each mind-body type is influenced by different tastes, there is a direct connection between what we hunger for and which mind-body characteristics predominate in our constitutions. On physical as well as emotional and mental levels, we may feel satisfied and therefore in balance, or unfulfilled and therefore lacking in a sense of well-being or equilibrium. From a weight- and stress-management perspective, modern Westerners are hungry people in literal as well as figurative terms, and Ayurvedic concepts may help us explore the relationship between what we hunger for (in the food we eat, in the thoughts we ingest, and in the actions we take) and our tendencies for overeating, overwork and overstimulation.

Excess Hunger

Excess hunger is demonstrated in Western culture in several ways, and not just with the consumption of food. As human beings, we feed ourselves on many levels of our existence. When we eat, most often we not only eat food

41

to keep the body alive, we use food as a source of enjoyment and nurturing. When eating feels compulsive or out of control, if the recollection of feeling deprived from previous dieting causes us to be anxious about being hungry, or when foods we crave are foods that don't make us feel well, the appetite becomes unbalanced and causes excess hunger.

We also feed our minds and spirits by the qualities of thoughts and actions we "ingest" every day. Our appetites for work, love, play, and rest may also be thrown out of balance, causing us excess and, therefore, imbalance. An Ayurvedic practice asks us to examine the connection between the "tastes" we ingest (both literally with food, and metaphorically with our actions and thoughts) and our resulting state of mind; by doing so, we begin to understand that feeding the body also feeds the intellect and emotions.

Conversely, what we feed our emotional and intellectual growth also affects our appetites for food and our ability to manage weight and stress. Using Ayurvedic principles, we may examine those characteristics and behaviors which are detrimental to a weight- and stress-management program from a more constructive, less self-criticizing view. As the cause of excess hunger is revealed, so the changes which lead to a more normal, relaxed appetite begin to show themselves. Solutions come more clearly when we view ourselves more kindly, giving our intelligence a chance to help balance our emotions and physiology.

One very prevalent example of aggravated Pitta (and deep hunger) in the West is our overconsumption of refined sugar. The West could be considered a Pitta-type society, because our values are often based on accomplishments and activities. As we have seen in chapter 3, people with a lot of Pitta in their constitutions focus their energy on accomplishing tasks, and naturally want "sweet" in their food (and also need "sweet" in their thoughts and actions), to turn down the pungent quality of a busy, perhaps overheated, day. In our culture, sweet is usually interpreted first as something we eat rather than something we think or do, and our poor, modern-day eating habits almost always represent a sweet food as something with refined sugar, and lots of it. Having an appetite is a normal function, and Pittas by nature have good appetites.

But people with Pitta require that their appetites be balanced by all tastes, including the more subtle sweet found in dairy, fruits, and vegetables, or their "sweet tooth" can get out of control. As most of us have experienced, it feels almost impossible to override cravings for sugar when sugar is consumed regularly—because refined sugar is in a powerfully concentrated form that obliterates the subtleties of the taste of sweet. Eating candy and other high-sugar sweets may send initial signals of relief from hunger by quickly sending blood sugar way up (that's the feeling of satisfaction) followed by a blood sugar low which sends signals for more sugar and excess carbohydrates; i.e., a continual cycle of hunger instead of a normal dance between hunger and satisfaction.

The prevalence of candida-related problems in the West is a byproduct of unsatisfied hunger and the influence of excess Pitta. When excess amounts of refined sugar, fermented foods (such as yeasted breads, vinegar, condiments, and alcohol), and moldy foods (such as mushrooms and hard cheeses) are consumed for extended periods of time, a condition called candida may result. This condition, sometimes also brought about or increased by an overconsumption of antibiotics, causes high yeast cultures in the digestive tract and destroys the "friendly" bacteria that helps us digest our food. The yeast, or "unfriendly" bacteria, turns the cravings for sugar way up, like a thermostat getting stuck on the "high" position, in order to "feed" itself. In a way, having a yeast overgrowth is like an allergy, as the body craves that which it does not need (i.e., the need for excess sweet), as a way to get us to pay attention and address the imbalance.

With candida, the mind sends a message to the body for sweetness, which in more metaphorical terms is saying that the body as well as the mind and emotions probably need large doses of sweeter, cooler, more astringent input to calm a fiery nature or slow down a superfast, high-pressure existence. Unfortunately, that signal is first heard by our physiology, which often gets an overwhelming signal for "sweet" food which cannot be controlled indefinitely by willpower (another Pitta characteristic). If we do not heed the deeper signal, the physical signal gets stronger and the cravings get worse. The immune system begins to weaken and our digestion suffers. Our less predominate mind-body characteristics (or sub-doshas) may also be affected, bringing further imbalance. It can become a viscious spiral difficult to stop, as anyone who has suffered from candida can tell you.

The Pitta tendency to overdo often causes weight and digestive imbalance, but by eating Ayurvedically and cooling down one's lifestyle, the hunger for sugar and excess carbohydrate is gradually replaced by the more natural sweet flavors found in fresh dairy, fruits, and vegetables, and the palate regains its ability to taste sweet in more subtler forms. The healthy palate also naturally sends our appetites signals for the carbohydrates found in vegetables and whole grains, thus bringing a feeling of satiation without the desire to ingest excess calories. In candida patients, yeast gradually dies back, reducing cravings and reinforcing healthy eating patterns. Reducing the amount of yeasted foods helps lower the yeast content in the digestive tract, which for most of us raised on processed foods and sugars is probably pretty high. Excess yeast compromises the body's immune system, destroys the body's ability to digest food properly, and leaves us sluggish and bloated—and craving sugar and excess carbohydrates as a way to "jumpstart" the body and mind into a state of energy. Eating refined sugar and excess carbohydrates eventually does not even bring a feeling of temporary relief, as the body reacts to the toxic side effects with headaches, feelings of lethargy and "spaciness," and digestive distress.

Many advocate extreme measures to get rid of sugar or yeast, but as with traditional diets that ask both body and mind to give something up, eventually the Pitta aspect of willpower cannot maintain the stress of resisting old, hard-to-give-up eating habits. Anything that sounds or feels extreme is functioning on excess Pitta power and will likely cause an additional imbalance in the sub-doshas. Shifting unhealthy eating patterns can be daunting, especially when they have been a part of our daily habits for so long. As we will discuss in chapter 6, we tend to resist something that indicates we are about to feel deprivation or uncomfortable cravings or sensations of withdrawal. "Pitta power," like sugar, is concentrated and powerful—that is to say, a little bit of

Pitta (like a teaspoon of sugar) goes a long way. Understanding the deeper hunger beneath cravings and deeper need for rest and play helps people influenced by excess Pitta to treat the source of the discomfort, and so eventually alleviate the hunger.

As a result of a hectic, modern environment, with overabundant choices of what to eat, what to do, and what to believe, the flip-side of our Western Pitta-like culture is Kapha excess. As a culture, the West (particularly in the U.S.) is hooked on sugar and overachievement. We are overdoers and overconsumers. What do we do when we're tired, exhausted, worn out, and fed up? We "numb out" and become Kapha couch potatoes, or become indifferent to the signals for hunger and nurturing we would normally receive in a healthy state. Being numb is like being in a black hole: all emotions and physical sensations combine at once to bombard the mind and body, resulting in a shutdown of the ability to make wise choices. We are sucked in to a feeling of inertia and apathy, and as the laws of science tell us, a body that becomes still tends to stay still. In other words, when we have arrived in a state of excess Kapha, it takes even more energy to get us out of it. Like a black hole—once in, it feels impossible to leave.

The irony is that in a healthy state, a person influenced by Kapha has great potential to not only maintain a moderate appetite but also an even approach to life which is less apt to be disrupted by life's ups and downs than a sensative Vata personality or a fiery Pitta temperament. The quality of Kapha offers a nurturing aspect that may be harnessed to develop good habits of personal self-care. Kapha-influenced people also love the various flavors of food, and Ayurvedic cooking directly appeals to the subtleties and varieties of tastes as found in herbs, spices, fresh produce, and whole grains. By nature, balanced Kapha types are naturally drawn to lighter foods such as salads and vegetarian dishes; they are also more apt to consume moderately proportioned meals because their enhanced ability to distinguish the different tastes in food gives them greater satisfaction (i.e., greater satisfaction per mouthful and, therefore, the ability to have less mouthfuls and still feel satisfied).

But just like Pitta, if Kapha is brought to excess, the natural indicator that says "I am satisfied" gets diminished, and the result is that the message sent gets garbled to "I can't seem to get enough." Healthy Kaphas like food, adventure, fun, and rest; imbalanced Kaphas move from natural moderation to "too much of a good thing is a good thing" mindset. The result: overeating beyond the point of feeling full, excess partying, and more naps and sleep-in mornings than workouts. Obesity is a Kapha imbalance, as is the overconsumption of consumer goods and planetary resources.

Mind-Body Combinations

Sometimes we take our ability to maintain balance for granted, but that aspect of our natures needs nurturing, too. It requires patience and consistency, both admirable Kapha traits. It benefits from the Pitta ability to harness the intellect to get to the root of the problem, and Vata's creativity and flexibility to invite change in. And since we all have these mind-body characteristics or doshas to varying degrees in our constitutions, it's important to be patient enough to discover those characteristics that truly influence us the most, and harness the constructive aspects of those doshas to create and maintain healthy, pleasing habits. In his book *Perfect Health*, Dr. Deepak Chopra gives excellent summaries of the sub-dosha combinations (Vata/Pitta, Vata/Kapha, Pitta/Vata, Pitta/Kapha, Kapha/Vata, and Kapha/Pitta) and their relationships to exercise.[4]

For the purposes of managing weight and stress, let's briefly look at the various combinations in terms of their constructive tendencies to affect appetite and handle stress. If a person is Vata/Pitta, chances are they like expending energy and have enough Pitta to help them keep an organized approach to diet and exercise as well as the ability to be create and solve problems (which helps reduce stress, as discussed in chapter 13). If a person is Pitta/Vata, they will tend to be more muscular and regimented, and their movement more purposeful, but they can get distracted from diet and exercise by work or too many goals. The key, then, is for Pitta/Vata people to keep self-nurturing a priority. Vata/Kapha will tend to be thin if in a balanced state but may tend to worry and put on weight if healthy habits are not established. If a person is Pitta/Kapha, the need to accomplish goals (such as exercise and diet goals) may be balanced by the natural Kapha desire to rest (and therefore avoid burnout and overintensity). Kapha/Vata people need to appeal to their desire for movement and ability to maintain a routine to avoid becoming heavy and inconsistent in their exercise; just as Kapha/Pitta people may engage their Pitta tendency to accomplish goals and use their even-tempered Kaph attributes to keep them from overdoing exercise or not initiate a regime.

As we begin to identify the constructive tendencies in our mind-body types, we may focus our energies on developing these qualities to assist us in our weight- and stress-management goals. Before outlining specific goals, however, let's explore the aspect of appetite further. Chapter 6 explores the deprivation caused by too much willpower-oriented dieting, as well as the deprivation we cause ourselves when we don't understand what our individual mind-body types need to feel satisfied on all levels. Chapter 7 delves into the deeper hunger often most prevalent behind eating imbalances; namely, the emotional hunger we cause ourselves when we ignore the need to feed our spirits.

The purpose of Ayurvedic Balancing is to create abundant, wise choices—a great contrast to the more Western approach to "deprivation dieting" and over-reliance on willpower and fear as motivators. As we identify all our hungers, and learn ways to satisfy ourselves on deeper levels, the motivator for personal growth moves beyond forceful intensity and avoidance of pain to a natural but conscious awareness of the desire for health. In short, as we balance our appetites, we unleash our natural ability to hear our needs and take care of them, in a constant dance (rather than a struggle) of the doshas or mind-body types to identify a hunger and feed it meaningfully. We become abundant, well-fed beings on all levels, and slowly but surely move away from our past feelings of insatiable hunger.

6

Dieting and Deprivation

The personal relationship that we develop with food builds up over time and reflects positive as well as negative experiences. In a healthy state, we have appetites to let us know when our bodies require food, and probably good memories and feelings associated with the consumption of food. We also have a highly sophisticated sense of taste, which helps us distinguish those flavors which are desirable for our particular mind-body configurations as well as gives us enjoyment while we eat. With the amount and variety of food available to people in the West, our culture could be considered a society of abundance, perhaps even of excess. Only a few generations ago, food was something a person had to work very hard for, and scarcity and lack of variety were commonplace. Now, with too many choices facing us, our inability to make healthy food choices often manifests as obesity, sluggishness, and digestive problems. Yet it's ironic that a culture so rich with food can be so obsessed with thinness, dieting, and the feelings of deprivation that dieting causes.

Our physiology is designed to store some fat in order to ensure the preservation of life; remember, we human beings have faced the possibility of starvation for most of our evolution, and many parts of the planet still suffer from lack of food. Modern medicine tells us that a woman's body naturally stores fat, especially during pregnancy, and too little body fat can interfere with normal bodily processes such as elimination, menstruation, and proper nerve functioning. But sedentary lifestyles, poor eating habits, and social definitions of beauty based on thinness create pressures for both men and women to store more fat than is healthy. And so we obsess with fat, and probably contribute to its increase because of our worry. As anyone who has ever been on a diet can tell you, the moment you decide to restrict calories, that's when you begin to feel deprived, even anxious, about getting enough food. In many people, particularly those influenced by Vata, feelings of nervousness trigger appetite, and so we probably tend to overeat both as a physical and a mental reaction to the feelings of deprivation that dieting causes.

Over time, a constant restriction of calories also plays havoc with our bodies, reducing metabolism and thus lowering the amount of calories needed to sustain basic functioning. A healthy body reflects a healthy appetite—for physical activity as well as food—and a person's metabolism is affected by the amount of energy expended as well as the amount of food consumed. We are meant to store some fat as energy reserve as well as lean mass which includes muscle, bones and organs; but if the ratio between lean-to-fat mass gets disrupted, the body often stores too much fat (in other words, it manifests a Kapha imbalance). This ratio between fat and lean tissue implies that in a healthy, fit state, the food that a person consumes will go primarily toward upkeep of lean mass and energy expenditure rather than to fat storage.

A person's metabolism is one of the primary factors in weight management; it is a mechanism, rather like a thermostat, which adjusts itself to the combined total of activity and food consumption. In a healthy state, a body's metabolism should be like a hot oven, ready to burn up calories and produce necessary fuel for energy expenditure. If a person restricts physical activity (especially fitness activities that sustain muscle mass) or adequate calories over a long period of time, the metabolism adjusts by lowering the amount of heat needed to burn fuel and produce energy. In other words, the higher the lean mass in a person (which is maintained by physical exertion and adequate calories), the higher the metabolism.[5] Conversely, the less a person eats and moves, the lower the metabolism; and the less a person wants to move, the more a person's body will store fat.[6]

A healthy goal, then, is to keep metabolism functioning well, so that we may eat a reasonable amount of food to satisfy our appetites and have enough energy to be active and feel vibrant. Looking leaner and feeling lighter are byproducts of this focus on metabolism. Unfortunately, most people approach their physical health and appearance from the outside first, focusing on how they look rather than laying groundwork to ensure a healthy lean-to-fat ratio (and metabolism), which allows for the proper functioning of muscles, organs, and thought. Restricting calories without maintaining proper physical activity will lead to some fat loss, but probably some loss of lean mass as well. Over time, however, a person's appetite (and the feelings of deprivation caused by calorie restriction) will probably override willpower, and a person will gain back weight—usually in the form of fat—making the person fatter than before the diet. This "yo-yo" dieting, with body weight going down and up, is often repeated in a chronic dieter, and the result is a metabolism which has naturally lowered itself (to preserve life) and thus shifted the lean-to-fat ratio in favor of fat storage, not the maintenance of lean body mass. It creates tremendous stress on the organs and systems of the body. Our physiology is designed to protect life, and prolonged caloric deprivation will increase the appetite as a way to increase fat and protect against starvation. Our physiology is not concerned with what we look like, it simply wants our bodies to live; and part of a healthy physiology is a healthy metabolism which thrives on proper exercise and nutritious food, resulting in a leaner, stronger, and lighter body.

Overcoming an increased or aggravated appetite caused by prolonged dieting is easier once we realize that we need to feed ourselves what our minds and bodies really desire, i.e., food, activity, and rest appropriate to the particular mind-body constitutions we have. Over time, constant dieting produces sluggishness of mind and body. The mind needs proper carbohydrate intake to function well, and the body's metabolism will slow down to move to a fat storage state, thus decreasing a person's desire to expend energy. Our emotions are affected, too, as the pleasure that food once gave us is now taken away by the concern and worry of restricting intake and avoiding specific foods. Eventually the body, mind, and spirit will rebel if food is viewed as a source of discomfort rather than as a natural way to enhance our feelings of being nurtured and well fed, resulting in imbalance.

Ayurvedic nutrition, on the other hand, is purposefully designed to enhance the feeling of well-being and satisfaction a person gets from food. As each mind-body type responds to appetite in a different way, knowing our tendencies in more objective Ayurvedic terms gives us more mindful ways to change our bodies and behaviors without unwittingly causing further imbalance and feelings of deprivation. Ayurvedic nutrition is designed to balance the appetite and reduce excess hunger, therefore creating a feeling of healthy abundance. Because Ayurvedic nutrition feeds the body at the level of taste (which, as we have seen in chapter 3, affects our state of being), it truly satisfies. And since a healthy body naturally wants to use metabolism to preserve lean mass, the natural mechanisms of appetite and energy are not distorted or suppressed.

Ayurvedic nutrition does not rely on willpower; rather, it appeals to a person's natural tendency in a healthy state to seek balance, which means that it is designed to satisfy a person's appetite on all levels, not just rely on calorie consumption as the primary means of comfort. Ayurvedic nutrition introduces a variety of tastes and textures, which create feelings of abundance; and being mindful of other ways to feed ourselves increases this feeling (and therefore decreases feelings of deprivation which trigger appetite). Balancing helps us expand choices to include food and activities that truly nurture and satisfy, and address deeper hungers, which may be triggering our appetites to aggravated levels.

7

ॐ

Emotional Hunger

By identifying and understanding our emotional connections to food and overaccomplishment, we may begin to get fed on other levels which include a variety of other nurturing practices which directly soothe the imbalance that often triggers food hunger or over-work. Nervous eating, which is a disrupting tendency of imbalanced Vata, may over time produce chronic conditions such as obesity and diabetes. Overwork, a Pitta tendency, supercedes our other needs to get enough rest and play. And eating from boredom or understimulation (Kapha in excess) also invites the palate to eat salt, sugar, and fat, because these particular qualities instantly bring a temporary physical sensation of stimulation or relief (but do not feed us at our deeper levels of hunger.)

Eating to numb loneliness and emotional emptiness is a subject covered extensively in *Love Hunger: Recovering from Food Addiction* by Dr. Frank Minirth, et. al.[7] Feelings of emotional emptiness lead to emotional pain, which is often anesthetized by food (sugar, fats, salt), overwork, or perhaps alcohol. The over-consumption of food only temporarily relieves the pain, and the undesirable physical changes lead to guilt, shame, self-hatred, and feelings of emotional emptiness. Creating a diversion from deeper problems by chronic overwork will also lead to mental, emotional, and physical fatigue. The never-ending cycle of emotional food consumption is a heart-breaking example of "underfed Vata," of a lack of (human) warmth and self-acceptance, of unmet fear and overwhelming emotional isolation. Chronic overwork without enjoying the fruits of our labors makes life too dry and asceptic, another Vata tendency to imbalance. The opposite of overeating is self-imposed starvation or anorexia, where excess Kapha leads to an indifferent rather than regular appetite, and the opposite of overwork is apathy and underachievement, also signs of Kapha imbalance. Often, when people who have been underfeeding themselves finally begin eating, the held-back hunger returns in a vengence, causing overeating and perhaps the "love hunger" cycle described above. And when people who have relied on overwork to distract them from their deeper needs finally hear those needs rising up, the overwhelming output of emotion, physical exhaustion, and mental confusion can truly play havoc with a person's work, relationships, and sense of balance and well-being.

Ayurvedically changing our habits away from addictive-type foods or addictive-style work habits is not a removal or a destruction or a deprivation, it is a recognition of an imbalance and a conscious endeavor to satisfy the "hunger" in a nurturing and restorative way. Often the lack of relaxation and sense of ease for Pitta, or the need for feelings of safety and warmth for Vata, or the desire for more satisfying stimulation of mind and body for Kapha are the causes of imbalance.

In Ayurvedic Balancing, comforting or soothing an aspect of our mind-body types that is out of balance is not a taking away of a comfort but rather an invitation to restore and rejuvenate and rebalance—to give our mind-body types the essential and truly satisfying comforts which they need to keep us healthy and happy. We all have Vata, Pitta, and Kapha qualities to varying degrees. The goal is to be ourselves in our best form, whether it be with intelligent but compassionate Pitta, an even-tempered and motivated Kapha, or a creative rather than fearful Vata. By Ayurvedically managing our weight and stress, we discover which of these mind-body qualities predominate, and then we learn to bring out our more constructive tendencies which are unique to our mind-body configuration. Just changing the body's appearance by typical dieting, or introducing a few Yoga classes in an overachieving lifestyle is often not enough—our minds and bodies tell us this through the demonstration of imbalance in the Vata, Pitta, and Kapha aspects which make up our constitutions. It's like treating a symptom but not looking deep enough at the habit to find the cause of the discomfort. These symptoms of imbalance will continue to tap us on the shoulder for attention, and if left unattended for too long, their messages can seem like wrecking balls crashing through our lives, demanding that we stop all else until we alter our course to a more balanced life. An Ayurvedic approach asks for balance on all levels, so a deeper, undiscovered imbalance does not derail all the effort expended to address a more noticeable one. In this way, we can be ourselves in a healthy and relaxed manner, so we don't have to struggle to be thin or more even-tempered or more motivated, so we may feel naturally relaxed yet energized.

Calming Hunger

Ayurvedic weight- and stress-management is not so much about decreasing undesired food intake or behavior as it is about creating an abundance of healthy and desirable choices that increases desire for health rather than masks a hidden hunger or imbalance. In conjunction, a Yoga practice (including both the physical exercise and meditation components) allows us to develop a clearer, more nurturing focus and energy while decreasing nervousness, inflexibility, and fatigue. This balanced approach to life allows for growth and change, for the healthy expression of emotions, appetites, and desires, and for the ups and downs of living in a changing body and changing world.

If you've experienced "crash diets" or even an eating disorder, most likely you still carry an adversarial relationship with food caused by the trauma of unhealthy eating patterns. Fad diets appeal to our lack of patience, and the underlying disbelief that we can approach food in a consistent, pleasurable, and healthy way. Usually, an eating disorder is an outward attempt to fix the unfixable, to be perfect (and therefore desired and loved) in a world that is telling you that for some reason, you aren't good enough as you are. Even if you haven't experienced an eating disorder, the need for perfection can still be driving you to overwork while leaving you feeling underfed emotionally. The striving for perfection, the overwhelming need to achieve and succeed and take care of or please everybody else, the lack of trust that comes from early messages of shame or inability to overcome failure, all these can lead to an empty emotional space which is too easily fed by imbalanced work habits or poor food choices, especially in a culture of fast food, stimulants, sugar, and too little time for rest, play, and self-care. The quality of Vata is by nature fragile: very creative and whimsical on the one hand, and fearful and shamed on the extreme other. If you have come to see yourself as less than worthy of good things because of your weight or other aspect of your self, then a seed of "hunger" has been planted. Human beings need to be wanted and nurtured—that's the Vata in all of us.

Often, compulsive work habits indicate other parts of ourselves that are not being fed. And if you find that food has become an overwhelming way to feed that emotional hunger, then food usually becomes the enemy. On the level of taste, junk food appeals to our desire for sweet and salty and the richness of fat. These qualities are part of a balanced appetite, and when a person's appetite is balanced, a little naturally goes a long way. If our constitutions are not in balance, the cravings for these snacks, sweets, fatty, and salty foods may become hard to resist because they create very compelling physical responses. Influenced by the particular combination of Vata, Pitta, and Kapha in each of us, we can become chronically "underfed" mentally, emotionally, or spiritually, and the need to restore balance to these qualities may come out through the expression of increased appetite for junk food or addictive eating and work patterns. In other words, an imbalance in deeper aspects of our being appears through the most readily available mechanism: appetite—in the form of hunger for unhealthy amounts of sugars, salt, and fats, or perhaps as an overgrown "appetite" for success, manifesting as compulsive goal achievement, which makes no room for rest or play.

Excess hunger may, if not addressed at its deeper emotional source, create further physical imbalance such as digestive problems, ulcers, sleeplessness, irritability, and excess weight gain—which often then reinforces the shame or guilt we may feel about our appearance, eating habits, willpower, or accomplishments. It is a vicious and unkind cycle, and a place that our emerging consciousness allows us to see, study, and ultimately leave behind.

Compulsive eating, overwork, excess caregiving of others, or inner torment as body weight goes up and down—lowering the immune system and draining us of self-esteem and emotional energy—may all lead to excess Kapha which numbs us and surrounds us with enertia. The good news is that this Kapha messenger may help us to slow down, truly hear the messages that the painful parts of our histories bring us, and then soothe the upset, fearful Vata that has been moaning for attention. Unconscious and compulsive patterns (or Pitta in crisis mode) may then gradually be replaced by consciously nurturing practices; in other words, the burning fire of over-achievement is cooled by the desire for a more balanced lifestyle that allows for other aspects of satisfaction besides work. These new patterns, which we slowly incorporate over time into a healthy belief system, allow us to interact with others without robbing us of our own abilities to nurture ourselves back to a feeling of well-being. Personal wellness then becomes more of a constant rather than illusive state.

These new patterns are not based on a fear of being discovered as imperfect—they are by nature forgiving, joyful, and well schooled from past hard knocks. They are both the once youthful voice and now wiser adult combining to give self-care and create the ability to feel safe, balanced, and flexible yet strong. When upset Vata (or fear) is untended for a great length of time, usually the fiery aspect of Pitta gets aroused to extreme levels to "prove" self-worth and cover the shame of fear, to survive in a confusing situation. Excess Kapha usually ensues, because no one can run on hyperspeed forever! Just as the pendulum has swung in one extreme (fear) and then the other (numbness), it can also find the center again (meaningful activity balanced with physical, mental, and emotional rest). This growing feeling of balance helps give us motivation to try new eating patterns or ways of looking at ourselves and our past; or perhaps incorporate a healthy exercise routine into a less difficult and self-criticizing lifestyle; or learn to appreciate the message of fear, so that we may assuage the discomfort we feel at deeper levels. When soothed, emotional hunger will eventually dissipate, lowering physical and mental hunger and increasing emotional and therefore physical and mental energy.

Remember, the goal of balancing is not to be perfect, or have perfect control of our world, because that is an illusion. What we can do, however, is lay cornerstones for healthier living by making individual lifestyle choices and small, accumulative changes with our well-being in mind. In other words, we may positively affect our state of mind on a day-to-day basis, eventually leaving us with a continued sense of well-being that does not get destroyed by life's ups and downs.

In a Yoga practice, a student over time may begin to view the various physical sensations and emotional reactions of doing the exercises or postures with a more objective view, noticing how his or her reactions contribute to a nurturing or a disruptive state of mind. The meditation aspect of Yoga allows the student to take the practice of poses or postures to a more metaphorical level, allowing for a greater insight and ability in sustaining a nurturing state of being. Yoga teaches us to move from different states of being—from feeling satiated to feeling empty, for example—more smoothly and with less anxiety. In this way, Yoga combines with its sister science, Ayurveda, to help us use our healthy desire for balance constructively, rather than unconciously relying on willpower, control, and underlying fears. Once we begin to identify our imbalances, we may then learn how to feed ourselves well on all levels of our being, compelled to seek balance because of the deep, satisfying comfort that nurturing ourselves brings. In this way, balancing becomes a self-sustaining mechanism, a natural desire to be well, and the opposite of struggle and failure.

8

What's Eating You?

As we've seen thus far in Part 2, calming excess hunger is not just about eating food; it's about recognizing and choosing that which sustains us as healthy, happy human beings. Intimacy and nurturing relationships, meaningful and rewarding work, and opportunities for self-care and personal growth are areas in which we "feed" ourselves our life experiences. Excess hunger in our lifestyles is easily brought on by a modern culture bursting with an overabundance of choices and not enough time or conscious ability to know which choices truly serve our needs. We tend to erode our personal foundations of well-being, even though we have an incredible choice of foods to eat, things to do and buy, and knowledge to assimilate, because *without a personal sense of self on a fundamental level it is easy to get overwhelmed by the overabundance of choice.* Discovering what is beneficial for our mind-body types is not always an easy task, as we are faced with the often difficult work of uncovering those circumstances and events which cause discomfort.

In *Care of the Soul,* Thomas Moore eloquently describes the learning process of the more spirited or soulful parts of ourselves which may dance to a seemingly illogical rhythm.[8] He explains that rationality—that part of us which wants to get from point A to point B in a straight and efficient line—does not always apply to personal growth, as the time we need to assimilate change is not readily governed by a preset, totally controllable timetable. Often our journeys to find comfort mean coming to know the discomfort we have created for ourselves. As Dr. John Welwood indicates in his book, wellness not only requires good food, exercise. and rest; it requires a "Journey of the Heart" as we seek to know what causes us to choose the lives we live and understand and assimilate the mechanisms of change—transforming "what's eating us" into food for the body as well as for our hearts and minds.[9]

Table 5 on the following page can help you begin to notice when you push yourself to your physical or emotional limits to the point that stress creates a trigger response to food. See if a drive for perfection causes you to be too hard on yourself and too critical of your accomplishments and efforts.

What makes you feel . . .	Satisfied or "full"?	Dissatisfied or "empty"?
In Your Work or Career		
Occupation or vocation:		
Family life:		
Other relationships:		
House/home maintenance:		
Education/Spiritual or personal growth:		
Fitness or exercise:		
While You're At Rest		
Meals/Why I eat:		
Particular foods I eat:		
Relaxation/Self-nurturing:		
Sleep patterns:		
When You Play		
Recreation/social activities/hobbies or pastimes:		

Table 5: **Identifying Hunger**

Can you describe or illustrate what hunger feels like to you?

_____

_____

_____

_____

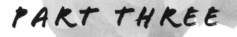

PART THREE

Calming
the Appetite

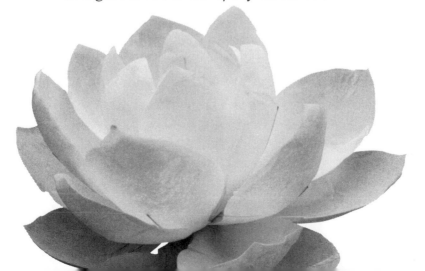

In my daily life
there are certain truths I must honor
certain joys I seek, certain ways of living
and if all are gathered with care and time
a spiralling future may continue to climb
My abundance may blossom
as I gather the truth of my riches . . .

9

ॐ

Satisfying Foods

In Ayurveda, the tastes in various foods may enhance or disrupt the ability of our mind-body types to maintain balance. As discussed in chapter 2, our physical state is directly connected to our minds and emotions, and eating specific foods may help reduce hunger, illness, and stress by appeasing prevalent imbalances. Amadea Morningstar's *Ayurvedic Cooking for Westerners* provides lists of foods for each mind-body type that are nurturing and soothing to that type.[10] Even though Ayurvedic cooking is vegetarian, Morningstar recognizes the challenge of introducing a vegetarian diet into our Western, meat-eating culture and includes animal products in her lists of foods. As you read through the following lists in Table 6, circle the foods you like, or would like to try. The foods you circle that fall under the two doshas or mind-body categories influencing you the most are the foods that are the most nurturing to your constitution.

Perhaps daunting at first, choosing foods that agree with (and therefore enhance the constructive qualities of) our mind-body types becomes a self-sustaining habit as we begin to feel the positive effects of our choices. The concept of Balancing expands our awareness of the variety of nurturing food choices, rather than focusing on restricting foods. In Part 3 we begin to create healthy, abundant choices. Sometimes what we find the hardest to change is that which we need the most, like a bodybuilder who only trains chest muscles (and so has a great looking set of "pecs") but who has no lower body to balance out the sculpted area on top. In Part 4, what we find difficult to change may become a series of little victories, building step by step a personal foundation of balance.

Food Type	Vata	Pitta	Kapha
Herbs & Spices	allspice	fresh basil*	allspice
	anise	black pepper*	anise
	asafoetida	cardamom*	asafoetida
	basil	cinnamon*	basil
	bay leaf	coriander	bay leaf
	black pepper	cumin	black pepper
	caraway	dill	caraway
	cardamom	fennel	cardamom
	cayenne*	mint, peppermint	cayenne
	cinnamon	neem leaves	cinnamon
	cloves	orange peel*	cloves
	coriander	parsley*	coriander
	cumin	saffron	cumin
	dill	turmeric	dill
	fennel	vanilla*	fennel*
	garlic	wintergreen	garlic
	ginger		ginger
	horseradish		horseradish
	mace		mace
	marjoram		marjoram
	mint, spearmint		mint, spearmint
	mustard seeds		mustard seeds
	nutmeg		neem leaves
	onion, cooked		nutmeg
	orange peel		onion
	oregano		orange peel
	paprika		oregano
	parsley*		paprika
	peppermint*		parsley
	poppy seeds		poppy seeds
	rosemary, saffron		rosemary
	sage savory		saffron
	tarragon thyme		sage

Table 6: **Recommended Foods** (*In Moderation **Occasionally)

Food Type	Vata	Pitta	Kapha
Herbs & Spices *(cont'd)*	turmeric vanilla wintergreen		savory tarragon thyme turmeric vanilla* wintergreen
Fruits	sweet fruits apricots avocado banana all berries cherries coconut dates figs, fresh grapefruit grapes kiwi lemons limes mango, ripe melons, sweet oranges, papaya peaches pineapple plums raisins, soaked rhubarb strawberries	sweet fruits apples, sweet apricots, sweet avocado berries, sweet coconut dates dried fruit, soaked grapes, sweet mango, ripe melons oranges, sweet pear persimmon pineapple, sweet* plums, sweet pomegranate prunes quince, sweet raisins watermelon	apples apricots berries cherries cranberries figs, dried mango, ripe peaches pear persimmon pomegranate prunes quince raisins strawberries*

Table 6: **Recommended Foods** (*In Moderation **Occasionally)

Food Type	Vata	Pitta	Kapha
Vegetables	acorn squash	acorn squash	artichoke*
	artichoke	artichoke	arugula
	asparagus	asparagus	asparagus
	bean sprouts	bean sprouts	bean sprouts
	beets	bell pepper*	beets
	butternut squash	broccoli	beet greens
	carrots	Brussels sprouts	bell pepper*
	cress*	burdock root	bok choy
	cucumber	butternut squash	broccoli
	daikon radish*	cabbage	Brussels sprouts
	fennel	cauliflower	burdock root
	garlic, cooked*	celery	cabbage
	green beans	Chinese cabbage	carrots
	leeks, cooked	collard greens	celery
	mung sprouts	cucumber	celtuce
	fresh corn	dandelion greens	chicory
	mustard greens*	endive	collard greens
	okra, cooked	escarole	fresh corn
	olives, black & green	fennel	daikon radish
	onion, cooked	green beans	dandelion greens
	parsnip, potato,	Jerusalem artichoke	eggplant*
	sweet pumpkin*	jicama	endive
	radish rutabaga	kale	escarole
	scallopini squash	leafy greens	garlic
	shallots, cooked	lettuce	green beans
	summer squash	mizuna*	horseradish
	watercress winter	mushrooms**	Jerusalem artichoke
	squash, yellow	okra	jicama
	crookneck squash	olives, black*	kale
	zucchini	bok choy	kohlrabi
		parsnips	leafy greens, all kinds
		peas	leeks
		potatoes, sweet	lettuce
		potatoes, white	mizuna
		radoccjop	mushrooms**
		rutabaga	okra
		scallopini squash	onions*

Table 6: **Recommended Foods** (*In Moderation **Occasionally)

Food Type	Vata	Pitta	Kapha

Vegetables *(cont'd)*		sprouts, all kinds
		snow peas
		summer squash
		Swiss chard
		winter squash
		yellow crookneck
		squash
		zucchini
			peas
			peppers
			potatoes, white
			radicchio
			radish
			scallopini squash
			shallots
			snow peas
			spinach
			sprouts, all kinds
			summer squash
			Swiss chard
			turnips* &
			   turnip greens
			watercress
			yellow crookneck/
			   zuccini

Grains	amaranth*
	oats, cooked
	rice, all kinds
	teff *
	wheat
	wild rice
		barley
		oats, cooked
		rice, basmati
		rice cakes
		rice, white
		wheat
		wheat bran
		wheat granola
			amaranth
			barley
			buckwheat
			corn
			granola, low-fat
			millet
			oats, dry
			oat bran
			popcorn
			quinoa
			rice, basmati, small
			   amount w/
			   peppercorn or clove
			rice cakes*
			rye
			teff
			wheat bran**

69

ॐ

Satisfying
Foods

Table 6: **Recommended Foods** (*In Moderation **Occasionally)

Food Type	Vata	Pitta	Kapha
Animal foods	chicken or turkey (white meat) duck & duck eggs eggs freshwater fish seafood	chicken or turkey (white meat) egg white* freshwater fish* rabbit shrimp*	chicken or turkey (dark meat) eggs, not fried or scrambled with fat rabbit
Legumes	beans (in moderation, soaked and well cooked): aduki black lentils mung red lentils soy cheese** soy milk soy yogurt** tepary tofu* tur dal urud dal	beans: aduki black black-eyed peas chana dal garbanzos khala chana kidney common lentils lima mung navy, white pinto soy products (flour*, powder**) split peas tempeh, tepary	beans (especially pre-sprouted): aduki black black-eyed peas chana dal garbanzos lima khala chana navy, white pinto red lentils soy milk, warmed* split peas tepary tofu, hot* tur dal
Nuts	In moderation: almonds black walnuts coconut Brazil nuts cashews coconut English walnuts hazelnuts macadamia nuts pecans pine nuts pistachios**	almonds, well soaked**	almonds, well soaked**

Table 6: **Recommended Foods** (*In Moderation **Occasionally)

Food Type	Vata	Pitta	Kapha
Seeds	chia flax pumpkin sesame sunflower	psyllium pumpkin* sunflower	chia flax* pumpkin* sunflower*

Sweeteners	barley malt syrup
	brown rice syrup
	fructose
	most fruit juices
	fruit concentrates
	raw honey
	maple syrup
	molasses
	sucanat
	sugar cane juice
		barley malt syrup
		brown rice syrup
		maple syrup
		fructose*
		sucanat*
		sugar cane juice
			raw honey
			fruit juice concentrates,
			    especially apple &
			    pear

Dairy	in moderation,
	    all fresh dairy:
	butter*
	fresh buttermilk
	raw cow's milk
	soft cheeses
	yogurt
	ghee
		unsalted butter*
		cottage cheese
		ghee
		soft cheeses**
		raw cow's milk
		ice cream
		sour cream
		fresh yogurt, diluted
		    1:2–3 parts with
		    water
			fresh goat's milk
			ghee* (clarified butter)
			diluted yogurt 1:4
			    parts or more with
			    water

Table 6: **Recommended Foods** (*In Moderation **Occasionally)

10

Becoming Well Fed

Learning to balance food habits Ayurvedically is a step-by-step process, best done in small "bites." As discussed in chapter 6, so often the word *dieting* conjures up feelings and memories of deprivation, which is a state of being that our beings will probably do the utmost to avoid! In Ayurvedic Balancing, we replace those food choices and habits that do not nourish and satisfy us with ones that do; in other words, we learn to seek a healthy abundance that asks us to eat great-tasting, satisfying food and get enough rest and relaxation from the hustle and bustle of modern life. When we begin to balance our mind-body constitutions, we start to nurture those aspects that may be aggravated and pay attention to those aspects and tendencies that often lead to a lack of well-being. By consciously feeding ourselves—on all levels, not just with food—we begin to bring out more constructive aspects that help us achieve our weight and stress management goals.

A typical Western fat-loss diet usually focuses on restricting food choice and limiting calories. As we have seen in chapter 7, our spirits are more likely to be motivated by abundance rather than limitation, and a restrictive type of diet by its very nature reduces motivation because it causes feelings of deprivation and emotional hunger. This kind of dieting relies on willpower, which is not a self-sustaining mechanism for behavioral change.

Eventually willpower breaks down, because a person's constitution will try to rectify the imbalance caused by overuse of this Pitta quality.

In chapter 5, we discussed the affects of Pitta imbalance manifested as an inflamed appetite, including the condition of yeast overgrowth called candida. Some Western approaches to the reduction of yeast in the digestive tract focus on reducing excess carbohydrates in an effort to "starve the yeast."[11] In *Ayurvedic Cooking for Westerners*, Amadea Morningstar outlines a gradual approach to the reduction of candida and suggests that *those foods we crave and therefore consume be reduced by increments of one-fourth the current level, to let these foods gradually lose their appeal.*[12] We cut back on the offending food or habit by one-fourth the amount, and when we feel comfortable with the new level, we cut back another fourth, and then again another fourth. As an example, if you eat a lot of spicy foods but are trying to reduce excess Pitta, you could try a more balancing and flavorful Ayurvedic recipe every third day, then eventually every other day, and finally have spicy foods occasionally as a treat. If you suffer from candida and have become used to eating yeasted breads but need to eliminate them from the diet, gradually introduce tortillas and flatbreads or crackers, eat fruit instead of candy, and try muffins sweetened by fruit (see recipes in chapter 12).

These newer food choices satisfy a healthy palate and help normalize appetite, which is fundamentally based on your mind-body type. As you cut back on the old habit, you replace that one-fourth with a new, more agreeable habit that feeds your mind-body type and reduces imbalance. This way, your body and emotional memories don't feel deprived, and change is gradually introduced in an acceptable, tangible way: your palate begins to regain its sense of taste by experiencing new and flavorful recipes and starts desiring foods that are nurturing and agreeable to your particular constitution. If cutting back on an offending food is difficult, then allowing your emotional and physical attachments to gradually be reduced introduces a healthy change in a more "digestible" manner. *The key to initiating the process of balancing is to gradually experience that changing to a more balanced way of eating will not only help reduce the undesired condition* (excess hunger or fat, candida, low energy, etc.), *but will feel truly satisfying* and, over time, will become a desirable and natural habit. It's important for us Westerners to accept the fact that most lasting change does not come overnight—a reality that our impatient Pitta culture tries to resist (and our Kapha imbalance tries to ignore). What reinforces positive change is a shift towards the belief that living a balanced life feels good, supported by actual experiences of making small changes and feeling their benefits (which is motivation by desire, not by willpower that is driven by fear or frustration).

Beginning Steps to Balanced Living

Rather than trying to change your habits into an Ayurvedic lifestyle overnight, consider the following suggestions, which may be introduced step by step, giving you time to assimilate not only the idea but to actually feel and internalize new habits:

1. *Start by eating more fresh fruits and vegetables*—a minimum of five servings or approximately two and one-half cups a day is a good start. If you are used to frozen vegetables and canned fruits, visit the produce section of your local supermarket more often and feast your eyes on the abundance of colors, smells, textures, and tastes. Freshly prepared food has more nutrients, vital energy, and flavor than frozen or processed food and is easily prepared. It doesn't take much time to steam or stir-fry fresh veggies, and fresh fruit is easy to take with you for a snack wherever you are. As you get used to eating more fresh produce, farmers' markets and organic food stores will seem like a natural progression in your increased desire for freshness and pesticide-free food.

How shall I increase my fruit and vegetable intake to 5 servings a day?

_____

_____

_____

2. If you "know what you're supposed to eat" but don't know where to start or can't get motivated to change your eating patterns, make it easy on yourself by cooking simple-to-prepare Ayurvedic recipes that have been especially designed and tested to nurture all constitutions. Try recipes included in chapter 12 of this book, or use a cookbook like *Ayurvedic Cooking for Westerners* by Amadea Morningstar. *Giving yourself thirty minutes a day to cook a great-tasting food is an achieveable goal,* and gradually incorporating Ayurvedic cooking into a daily routine lets the tastebuds lose their dullness to all the tastes so that flavors come alive and a little sweet feels like a treat. It may feel intimidating at first, but soon your meal preparation may become a rewarding part of the whole experience of using food to nurture, to satisfy, and to keep the body fit and healthy (and a great way to spend quality time with others). If the idea of cooking new recipes (or cooking at all!) feels overwhelming, begin simply by trying one new Ayurvedic recipe a week and build up your new food habits gradually.

Review the foods you circled in the list of recommended foods (in Table 6 from the previous chapter) and write down some new food choices you would like to buy on your next trip to the market.

3. What foods do I crave or "have to have" to feel satisfied? Are these foods disruptive to my health-, weight-, and stress-management goals? If so, how? What new food choices may I make which agree with my mind-body type?

_____

_____

_____

_____

Foods I Crave	Disruptive Aspects	New Balancing Choices
Breads, starches, cereals:		
Desserts and sweets:		
Spices, fats, and salt:		
Red meat and dairy:		
Fermented condiments:		
Alcoholic beverages:		

4. In his book *Perfect Health,* Deepak Chopra gives several suggestions for increasing the satisfaction we get from food.[13] He recommends we:

- Eat in a calm atmosphere, avoiding meals when upset

- Sit down to eat a meal, refraining from talking with a full mouth or gulping food down so that the body has time to receive signals that physical hunger is being satisfied

- Take a few moments after the meal to sit quietly and appreciate the meal to help the food absorb into physical as well as emotional systems

■ Eat freshly cooked meals which include all six tastes, and if used to big meals or portions, gradually reduce the size of the meal so that one-third to one-quarter of the stomach is empty to aid digestion. (Rule of thumb for portions: one meal is approximately two handfuls.)

If you love to eat and find your appetite for good food is leading you to an increased waistline, finding a balance between the tendency to "splurge and party" and eating satisfying and lighter meals is a gradual shift, begun by noticing existing habits.

How do I eat meals now? Are there any changes I would like to make?

_____

_____

_____

_____

5. An excellent practice before a meal is taking time for ten minutes of quiet sitting. This is good for all mind-body types as it helps calm nervous eating (Vata imbalance), eating when upset or tense (Pitta imbalance), and the tendency to numb our senses by overeating (Kapha imbalance).

What other ways would I like to enjoy relaxation time in my daily life?

_____

_____

_____

_____

6. Getting fed in other ways besides food also decreases the likelihood that eating (or other activity that poorly "feeds" you) becomes the most significant way to "feel full": Get in touch with the "sweet things" in life that are readily accessible and give happiness. Some possibilities include spending quality time with loved ones; setting aside time for a good book or hobby; enjoying some everyday pampering like a foot massage, comforting bath or shower, quiet moments of sunshine, beauty (a walk in a garden, a favorite magazine, music); laughter (a funny movie, playing a game, a good joke), and physical exercise.

What comforting and enjoyable activities currently give me happiness? What other activities would increase my daily enjoyment of life?

_____

_____

_____

_____

7. The self-critic in us can be useful to urge us to better ourselves, but used habitually, we may begin to erode our emotional and even physical well-being. Do you habitually ask yourself to accomplish to the point of fatigue?

When do you push yourself to emotional or physical exhaustion? Conversely, what motivates you to achieve goals?

_____

_____

_____

_____

11

ॐ

Ayurvedic Cooking

One easy way to begin eating foods more nourishing to your particular mind-body type is to cook recipes found in many of the books listed in the Appendices section of this book. One very good book for beginners trying to introduce Ayurvedic cooking into a Western lifestyle is *Ayurvedic Cooking for Westerners* by Amadea Morningstar. It contains many great-tasting and easy-to-prepare recipes that are primarily sattvic or balancing to all mind-body types, and shows you how to cook not only for yourself but for other people with different constitutions. Morningstar, who uses many ingredients we are familiar with to make easy to prepare dishes, takes the guesswork out of how to select foods which appeal to particular mind-body types while introducing our palates to new and interesting spice-herb combinations and flavors. In addition, chapter 12 contains recipes I have created to help you introduce your palate to a variety of seasonings, grains, vegetables, and lighter protein sources; it also includes a seven-day menu and shopping list to help get you organized and started. As you shift your habits, eating meals with fresh produce becomes quite enjoyable.

Some Tips for Cooking Ayurvedically

1. Ideally, food should be prepared and consumed on the same day; however, I believe it would be better to cook fresh food the evening before and take it

to work the next day rather than missing a meal or eating nutritiously empty or aggravating food. To save time, Morningstar encourages use of a pressure cooker for cooking legumes, or soaking and then cooking them overnight in a slow cooker. Also, it takes about thirty minutes a day to cook an Ayurvedic main meal, and taking time to prepare and eat good food introduces a welcome pause in a busy day while re-aclimating the senses to the notion of self-care. Moving toward creating a balance between "downtime" and "busy-ness" greatly reduces the urge to overeat or eat food which aggravates our constitutions, and the planning, preparation, and consumption of balanced food can become truly comforting. Sometimes it feels more compelling to flop down on the sofa after a long day and microwave a frozen dinner—we all have those days. Like acquiring any new skill, cooking Ayurvedically takes some time and patience but eventually it feels desirable, normal, and easy (and chopping a few vegetables a day really is easy!).

2. Some Ayurvedic recipes may seem rigid at first, such as the preferred use of only fresh (raw, then boiled) cow's milk, clarified butter (ghee) instead of margarine or salted butter, or vegetarian ingredients. Allow yourself time to adopt these principles as they feel right for you. Remember, finding one's balance doesn't imply finding perfection, and the goal is to gradually change habits and eating patterns to bring health and happiness. So if you can't find raw cow's milk, use the organic, pasteurized kind more sparingly and introduce rice, soy, goat, and nut milks into your diet. With a little practice ghee is easy to prepare, and many of the recipes call for a variety of cooking oils which give great flavor variations while letting you watch cholesterol levels. If you're not used to vegetarian meals or find that you function better with some meat, fish, or poultry in your diet, add some of these to your shopping list while trying some of the recipes in their vegetarian form. Over time, you may find your palate changes and that you prefer eating in this lighter but satisfying way.

3. If you have concerns about reducing your appetite and food portions, using Ayurvedic recipes consistently will quickly "wake up" your taste buds

and help give you feelings of satiation and satisfaction (which in the past might have meant extra-large portions or extra amounts of sugars, salts, and fats). These balanced recipes satisfy hunger more easily, naturally curbing your appetite and allowing you to stop "counting calories" and weighing food portions. This way you create abundance, not deprivation.

4. Buying and preparing food may be unnerving if food has become the enemy from years of frustration with previous "dieting" or experiences with an eating disorder. Perhaps meal preparation and consumption for just oneself feels lonely. Sometimes it feels easier to avoid food (or not cook at all and grab a quick meal) than to face the hunger that dieting has caused. That deeper sense of hunger, that fear that there will not be enough willpower to resist candy, fatty foods, and other quickly satiating but unbalancing foods (and underneath, that fear of not feeling full and satisfied and comforted) sometimes keeps us from learning new skills to "calm the beast" of hunger that seems to rule us. Give these changes time! If cooking is new to you or seems too overwhelming, like an obligation or a chore that makes you feel tired or lonely, try for a few balancing recipes a week and perhaps give yourself permission to spend some time self-nurturing in other ways. Although it's not an open invitation for resistance to change to stop you from moving in a healthy direction, sometimes it takes time to examine the resistance to cooking Ayurvedically, before the desire to nurture one's self with healthy food practices brings motivation. Just stay with your process of personal growth, and in time you will know when it's right to make a change.

5. In Ayurvedic cooking, organic produce is preferred over produce grown with pesticides; yet if cost or availability are factors, know that you are still eating more healthily by consuming more "live foods" such as fresh supermarket fruits and vegetables. You might consider growing a backyard vegetable garden or herbs in a window box as a hobby and as a contribution to your preparation of food, or shopping at a farmer's market. Getting in touch with fresh produce at its source extends your satisfaction from and appreciation of food. Also, find a good health-food store in your area

where you can stock up on spices, herbs, grains, seeds, nuts, and legumes. These items, as well as fresh produce, give you lots of bang for your vegetarian buck, and are often less expensive than meals with meat.

6. Include supportive family and friends in your experimentation with these new recipes. It is important that you create a supportive environment for learning new habits, such as having enough time to eat a balanced meal during the day and sharing your food experience with others. Relationships or situations at home or work that are unsupportive of your desire to live in a balanced way often create roadblocks to creating new habits. When your desire is blocked, the result is frustration. The third section of this book examines the process of working with imbalance and skills you may acquire to support your desire to cook, eat, and live in a more balanced way.

7. In Ayurvedic cooking, meals usually consist of a light breakfast, a main meal, and a lighter evening meal. Suggestions for a lighter meal include: a salad bar and baked potato at restaurants; a cooked grain such as rice, millet, quinoa, or pasta with steamed veggies and tofu, nuts or seeds; fresh fruit for snacking; cooking extra portions of the main meal of the day to be eaten in the evening.

8. Reducing the amount of yeasted bread in our Western diets may feel difficult at first, because we have limited our palates in the West to mainly wheat, and we have become unimaginative when it comes to eating grains. Included in this chapter are recipes for easy to prepare muffins and suggestions for a variety of bread alternatives. The muffin recipes help you explore the tastes of new grains while still feeling satisfied by "bread," and they use fruits and fruit juices instead of sugar for sweetness to help reduce dependence on refined sugar. Once your palate becomes able to recognize the more subtle forms of sweet, you may find that traditional muffins are just too "sugary!"

9. In chapter 12 I have also included a few of my own recipes for you to try, as well as a seven-day menu and shopping list to help get you started. I

hope it doesn't take you as long as it took me to explore new recipes: I owned Morningstar's book for over a year before I actually used it! But then again, I had a lot of issues to work through around eating and hunger, and I felt I had only enough stamina to deal with my emotional issues first. (I am happy to say that her book is now a well-worn, well-marked source of great meals at our house!) What I didn't know—or perhaps really trust or believe—is that Ayurvedic cooking is not very difficult (especially with the help of such books as Morningstar's).

I also didn't trust the fact that eating Ayurvedically actually reduces appetite; but finally I reached a point in my growth that allowed me to let go of my need to use willpower alone to control my hunger. It was scary to trust that my appetite would normalize without counting calories. But ultimately, it has been a very rewarding experience, freeing me from the stress of deprivation dieting. Now when I cook for family and friends, they love all the fresh vegetables, different grains, flavorful herbs, and satisfying tastes. Little do they know that they are getting a taste of balance with each bite—and it doesn't even hurt a bit!

Vegetarian or Not Vegetarian: Is That Really the Question?

For me, switching from an overconsumption of yeasted bread to the inclusion of a broader variety of grains was a piece of cake compared to going from a lifelong meat-eater to becoming a vegetarian. Feelings of deprivation and restriction collided with other aspects such as convenience, belief systems and habits; after all, it's a big deal to change one's way of eating . . . or is it?

A few years back, I became a vegetarian for four years, eating (as one friend put it) "no cows, pigs, or chickens." I did so because I was heavily into Yoga and meditation, doing a lot of personal growth work and sorting out all kinds of emotional and physical questions—unravelling my own personal "ball of yarn" so I could create a clearer, healthier identity and lifestyle. I was just starting to learn about Ayurvedic nutrition but resisted it because of all the many emotional entanglements I had with food. Looking back, I realize that I made those four years very hard in terms of nourishing my constitution, because I had a hard time trusting that eating Ayurvedically could help me deal with my struggle to become a happy and satisfied person. Intellectually, I believed in the concept. I guess I didn't believe in my ability to apply this concept to my confused life, and was afraid of losing control.

An Ayurvedic approach to nutrition has now become more satisfying and realistic, but it wasn't always that way. Much of my vegetarian practice at that time in my life was focused on increasing my spiritual existence, and as David Frawley discusses in his book *Yoga and Ayurveda: Self-Healing and Self-Realization,* often an ascetic approach to food is good for creating a greater awareness of mind, but not so good for creating physical balance.[14] For example, as part of a Yoga meditation practice, fasting may cause heightened awareness, but it may also cause the more delicate aspect of Vata to become imbalanced, and often Westerners like me who tried to maintain a vegetarian lifestyle for spiritual reasons end up struggling to override feelings of deprivation and emotional hunger that limiting food intake or choice may cause.

As Frawley explains, sometimes these two sister sciences are at odds, even though both aid in personal growth. The meditative aspect of Yoga is more focused on gaining a clearer sense of one's spiritual self and may supercede the physical needs of the body, whereas Ayurveda is a very medicinal science, aimed at bringing physical well-being through the proper intake of food. It has taken me years of practice to not only intellectually comprehend but also physically and emotionally experience the great commonality between the two sciences; namely, that my spiritual growth can move into my day-to-day existence and include the nurturing of my physical health and fitness.

From the point of view of abundance, I believe we are meant to evolve into caring and conscious human beings who use intellect as well as emotions and the physical world to expand our understanding and nurturing of self and others. Both Yoga and Ayurveda can be very introspective, requiring the student to ask intricate and involved internal questions—as well as worldly, building a sense of community and commonality through a shared experience of physical, mental, and emotional hunger and nourishment. When I first became vegetarian, I was seeking to feed my spiritual hunger, as that was the appetite in me that raged the most. My Yoga and meditation practice has aided me in the task of creating more understanding of self, and now I find that my practice of balancing allows me to manifest that understanding into a daily practice of self care. Studying the principles of Ayurveda helped me expand this concept of balancing—to feed myself on all levels, therefore creating enough abundance in me so there would be something more to give to others that enhanced rather than depleted my life. After years of intense self-scrutiny and tearing down old ideas of what I thought was me, and learning patience so I could learn new life skills, I have become better equipped to feed myself that which I need. More specifically, I find that a vegetarian approach to eating is more appealing now that I have begun to address the imbalances in my lifestyle that affect my sense of well-being and therefore my appetite.

When I am overworked, or fearful, or lethargic, my appetite shifts to a heavier diet as a way to compensate for the physical, mental and emotional strain. When I make more conscious choices about my lifestyle, my hunger eases, and I don't need to eat as much, overdo as much, and struggle as much to feel satisfied. My focus then shifts from survival of self to meaningful participation in the world. It shifts from feeling hungry to noticing the hunger around me, and wondering what I can do to create more abundance internally so that it naturally overflows. But this process takes time, and the acceptance of hunger.

After four years of vegetarianism, I began to eat meat and chicken again, and felt I needed it. I was ready to address some really tricky hungers: the aftermath of an eating disorder, the overgrowth of intestinal yeast (which made me crave sugar and excess carbs), and a stressful career, which adversely affected my health and fitness. I finally let myself feel the "hungers" that my previous lack of understanding had created, trusting the Ayurvedic premise that in time my appetite would normalize as I learned how to feed myself on all levels of my being. I let my appetite be what it was—in transition. In other words, I let my ball of yarn unravel and let go of willpower as the main force behind my actions.

Slowly I was able to focus on feeding myself well, but there were many moments when I ate too much meat, sugar, and junk food; when I worried about that which I could not control; when I pushed too hard and paid for the subsequent physical fatigue and emotional and mental exhaustion. I've had to make some hard choices throughout this process: how to earn a living that could allow a healthier me to consistently thrive; how to maintain a nurturing spiritual practice in a modern world of nonstop achievement; how to reconcile my lifelong taste for meat with a fundamental Yogic principle of bringing no harm to living beings (and the growing awareness that a vegetarian lifestyle puts less strain on dwindling planetary resources). Whew! Changing my diet back to vegetarian seemed like a real pain.

That is, it was painful until I started to feel in balance. When I decided that I would rather be healthy than stressed (which gave me the courage to shift my career), I began to enjoy the people, things, and environment in my life more, and I didn't seem to need as much. Not to say that financial health is not important; in fact, it is a fundamental way we take responsibility for ourselves. But how I was to earn a living was the question I finally started to address, using the desire for balance as a signpost for change. Without the stress of doing something that no longer served, my ability to feel kind, peaceful, and worthy began to return, and I realized I was learning to feed my emotional emptiness with compassion, rather than cover it up with accomplishment and fear. I began to feel that not hurting myself and others was a primary objective, because I began to enjoy the feeling of not being such a hurt and wounded human being. My belief system began to shift out of desire (not a sense of duty) toward the Yoga principle of nonviolence that denounces the consumption of animals. I realized that shifting toward vegetarianism was a lifestyle choice that for me was incremental and not perfect. The turning point was when I realized that I was spending less time worrying about trying to do the right thing, i.e., be perfect, and more time focusing on improving my life in small, tangible, and meaningful ways. As I came to believe that eating less meat and trying more vegetarian meals agreed with my desire to feed myself well, my belief system shifted my appetite to want meat even less, and work even more consistentanty to give myself plenty of rest, nurturing, and clarity to maintain this more peaceful, i.e., less hungry, state.

It's tricky being vegetarian in our society. It's a lifestyle that cannot be forced on you simply because you think "it's the right thing to do" or because "it will bring enlightment." In time, you may grow to believe these things. But before you do that, you have to face your hungers. Work through them. Grow out of them. Get help and seek kindness. And let your appetite finally bring you where you need to be. In whatever way you work to identify and reduce a "hunger"—whether physical, or mental, or emotional—you are moving in a direction of self-nurturing and balance. If you keep moving in that direction long enough, surviving all the ups and downs and curveballs that your inquiries throw at you, you'll get to a place of reduced hungers on many levels. Most likely, you'll see yourself becoming "lighter," reducing bit by bit the excess weight of unmet fears and needs.

Bringing about balance can be painful at times. In my case, I think I've learned a lot in my journey to seek wellness, but I think I hurt myself a lot through my ignorance. I have learned that there are skills we can all learn and practice which help our process of personal growth along, and Part 4 of this book discuss specific ways you may expand your self-nurturing skills. Lastly, Part 5 outlines the cornerstones of Balancing so that you may create a truly personalized foundation for well-being.

12

ഘ

Balancing Recipes

Even if your focus is not a weight-management program, eating Ayurvedically can give you an expanded sense of abundance in your diet, and in your life. Often we get too busy or preoccupied with other things and unwittingly narrow our choices of flavors and textures in our meals. As you begin to consider Ayurvedic cooking, the seven-day Main Meal Menu, complete with recipes, is an easy way to explore a wide variety of herbs and spices, grains and legumes, nuts and seeds, and various kinds of protein sources. Also included is a recipe for nonyeasted muffins and tips for alternatives to bread. Great taste is at your fingertips—what are you waiting for? Have fun!

Each meal offers a different set of flavors, indicated by area of influence. While these meals may not be strictly Ayurvedic, they are an easy step in that direction, and a great way to introduce your palate to lighter, more flavorful meals that use less animal protein and greater variety of herbs and spices. All Main Meal recipes make four servings and may be easily reduced by half.

Day 1: Mexican Fiesta

Avocado-Pepita Salad, veggie burgers or Cilantro Turkey Burgers, Millet with Black Bean Salsa

Day 2: Oriental Stir-Fry

Cashew-Ginger Stir-Fry or Sesame-Cilantro Stir-Fry

Day 3: Italian Delight

Oregano-Tomato Green Beans with Onion-Pecan Quinoa and a Mixed Green Salad

Day 4: Mediterranean Brunch

Vegetable Three-Bean Salad with Potato-Broccoli Omelet

Day 5: Southern Feast

Black-Eyed Peas, Basil Potatoes, Spiced Beets and Greens, Rosemary Okra, Summertime Squash

Day 6: California Cool

Wild Rice Salad, Tarragon Green Beans with Almonds

Day 7: Hawaiian Express

Pineapple-Ginger Stir-Fry with a touch of curry; served plain or with brown or white rice

MEXICAN FIESTA

Avocado-Pepita Salad

Salad greens

> 8 cups mezclun mix or your favorite lettuces plus jicama slices (optional)
> ½ cup raw pumpkin seeds (pepitas)

Dressing

> 1 ripe avocado
> ½ cup cilantro
> 2 tsps. lemon or lime juice (or more, depending on taste)
> 1 small clove garlic, minced
> 2 tsps. Bragg Liquid Aminos (unfermented soy sauce, available at health-food stores)
> 1–2 tbsps. apple juice

Wash greens. Blend dressing ingredients in blender or food processor, using apple juice to get dressing to desired consistency. In a small skillet, roast pumpkin seeds (without oil) on high heat for about one minute, until seeds start to pop. Pour dressing onto greens and sprinkle with the toasted seeds. Note: the toasted pumpkin seeds give a very hearty flavor to salads and are great as snacks.

Cilantro Turkey Burgers

> 1 lb. ground turkey
> 1/2 cup cilantro, chopped
> 2–3 green onions, chopped
> 1/3 cup oats
> 1 egg or 2 egg whites
> Bragg Liquid Aminos (unfermented soy sauce)
> salt and pepper to taste

In medium-sized mixing bowl, combine egg, oats, and 1 tbsp. Liquid Aminos. Allow the oats to soak, about 10 minutes or so. Add cilantro and onions, mix thoroughly, adding salt and pepper if desired. Shape into patties and sauté in a little olive oil, or grill, until done. Note: Add a little more Liquid Aminos while cooking, to get a nice brown color. Since the patties are lean, they will tend to fall apart if you shape them too thin. For those who don't like a lot of cilantro, reduce the amount as your taste buds indicate. This is a very quick recipe, with lots of flavor.

Millet with Black Bean Salsa

1 cup millet
1 cup black beans
1 ripe tomato, cut into small pieces (or 6–8 cherry tomatoes, quartered)
1/4 cup cilantro
2 tbsps. chopped red or green onion
1/2 cup raw or cooked sweet corn kernels, removed from cob
1 tbsp. lime
1/2 cup plain yogurt
1/4 cup olive oil
2 tbsps. apple juice
salt to taste

Cook beans in water until done, soaking if possible a few hours or the night before. Rinse millet in water half a dozen times to remove soapy residue, using a strainer to catch the millet as you empty the water. Cook the rinsed millet in 2 cups water (and salt, if desired) until done, about 25 minutes. While millet is cooking, chop tomato, cilantro, and onion and place along with corn in medium sized bowl. In blender (or small bowl using a wire whisk) mix lime juice, yogurt, and olive oil; if dressing is too tart, add apple juice. If you want this to be a warm side dish, add chopped vegetables, black beans, and dressing to millet as soon as it is done and serve immediately; if you want to serve it as a salad, wait until the millet is cooled before adding the vegetables and dressing. Note: for a little "kick," try adding 1 teaspoon chopped green chili. Also, if you don't care for millet, you can use 2 cups cooked pasta shells.

ORIENTAL STIR-FRY

Sesame-Ginger Stir-Fry

1 cup each:
  bok choy
  broccoli flowerets
  sweet red pepper slices
  snow peas
  spinach leaves, torn into bite-sized pieces
  (or other vegetables—preferably without mushrooms—like chopped
     celery, bean sprouts, water chestnuts, and asparagus)
1–2 tsps. freshly grated ginger root
1 clove garlic, minced
1–2 tbsps. unfermented soy sauce (Bragg Liquid Aminos)
2 tbsps. toasted sesame oil
1 tbsp. brown rice or other flour
1/4 cup raw, hulled sesame seeds
1/3 cup chopped cilantro
cooked rice or bean thread noodles

Sauté the vegetables, garlic, and ginger root on medium high in toasted sesame oil; add 1 tbsp. Liquid Aminos when vegetables begin to sound "dry" as the oil cooks off, and enough water until vegetables are done. Cook the vegetables until they are tender-crisp—try not to overcook. Put the other tablespoon of Liquid Aminos into a small jar along with the flour and a little water, put cap on tightly and shake until flour is absorbed into the liquid. Turn heat to low, add flour mixture, and stir until sauce thickens. You may want to add more water or Liquid Aminos until you reach the desired consistency. In a small skillet, toast sesame seeds on high heat for about one minute until seeds start to pop. Sprinkle seeds onto vegetables, garnish with freshly chopped cilantro leaves, and serve with hot rice or cooked bean thread noodles (follow directions on the package).

For cashew variation:
Replace sesame seeds with 1/3 cup raw cashew pieces and replace the flour with 2 tbsps. cashew or almond butter, mixed with 1 tbsp. soy, 1 tsp. lime and 1–2 tbsps. apple juice. This will give the dish a richer, nuttier taste. For even richer taste, add coconut milk (lowfat version is available at health-food stores) to vegetables while they are cooking, instead of water; or cook it with rice, replacing 1 cup water with 1 cup coconut milk.

For extra protein:
You may sauté 8 ounces cubed tofu, chicken breast, or shrimp with the oil and garlic for a few minutes, and then add the vegetables and cook until done.

ITALIAN DELIGHT

Oregano-Tomato Green Beans

4 cups green beans, cut or snapped into one-inch pieces
1 cup cherry tomatoes, sliced into halves
1 clove garlic, minced
1/4 cup fresh oregano leaves, finely diced
1 tsp. unsalted butter or ghee (clarified butter)
1 tbsp. olive oil
salt and pepper to taste

In a medium-sized skillet, sauté the beans and garlic in the butter and olive oil on medium-high heat; add oregano and tomatoes when the oil has cooked off and vegetables sound "thirsty." Turn heat down to low, cover and simmer until beans are tender, adding water if necessary. Note: If you have a vegetable garden, and the beans and tomatoes start ripening all at once, this recipe helps you gobble them up in style. For flair, you can add 1/2 cup cooked garbanzo beans and 1/4 cup sliced black olives.

Onion-Pecan Quinoa

1 cup quinoa
2 cups of water
2 small or 1 large green onion, chopped
1/3 cup pecan pieces
salt and pepper to taste

In medium saucepan, rinse the quinoa half a dozen times to remove soapy residue. Cook in 2 cups water, uncovered, bringing to a boil. Then covering with lid, cut heat to low and cook for 15 minutes; add salt and pepper, onion, and pecan pieces. Continue to cook until all liquid is absorbed and quinoa grains are soft and plump. For added flavor and richness, you can add a little olive oil or butter/ghee when you add the nuts and onion. Note: Quinoa is a grain high in protein. The pecans add protein as well as a nice, sweet flavor.

MEDITERRANEAN BRUNCH

Vegetable Bean Salad

  1 cup dried white beans
  1 cup apple juice
  1 tbsp. diced red onion
  1/2 tsp. coarsely ground black pepper
  2 cups chopped vegetables (carrots, broccoli, zuccini work well)
  2 tbsp. olive oil
  1 clove garlic, minced
  1 tbsp. lemon juice
  1/4 cup each fresh basil and parsley
  salt to taste

Soak beans in medium saucepan for two hours or overnight. Drain beans and add apple juice, onion, pepper, and enough water until liquids cover the beans by 2 inches. Cook beans until tender, about 45 minutes. While beans are cooking, dice vegetables and garlic and sauté in 1 tbsp. olive oil until the green beans are tender-crisp (you may need to add some water and "steam" the vegetables a bit until the green beans are done). Let vegetables and beans cool, and mix with 1 tbsp. olive oil, lemon juice, basil, parsley, and salt if desired. Note: For exceptional color, use purple ruffled basil. You may also add other raw vegetables such as diced sweet red pepper or grated carrot for a crunchier texture.

Potato-Broccoli Frittata

9 egg whites and 3 whole eggs, whisked together
1 cup raw potatoes, diced
1 cup chopped broccoli (green peas, zuccini, and sweet red pepper
    work well too)
1 large or 2 small green onions, finely sliced
1 clove garlic, minced (optional)
1/4 cup fresh oregano, chopped (or 1/2 tsp. dried oregano leaves)
1 tsp. fresh rosemary leaves, finely chopped (or 1/2 tsp. dried leaves)
1–2 tbsp. Liquid Aminos (unfermented soy sauce)
1 tbsp. olive oil
salt and pepper to taste

In large skillet over medium high heat, sauté onion (and garlic if desired), potatoes, and rosemary in olive oil until vegetables start to brown. Add Liquid Aminos and enough water to "steam" potatoes until they are tender-crisp, adding more water as it cooks off, if necessary. Add broccoli (or other vegetables, if desired) and oregano. Reduce heat to medium-low and slowly pour beaten eggs on top of vegetables. To keep frittata from becoming too brown on the bottom, add a little water around the edges of the frittata for steam, and cover with a lid or a piece of foil. You may have to add additional water as the frittata cooks. The frittata is done when knife inserts cleanly into center (allow 10–15 minutes for the eggs to cook). Note: for added flavor, add a couple of slices of soy cheese to the top of the frittata a few minutes before it's done, or some fresh salsa, or both!

A SOUTHERN FEAST

This meal may take a bit longer, but it is well worth it!

Black-Eyed Peas

> 2 cups fresh or 1 cup dried black-eyed peas
> 1 large bay leaf
> 1 clove garlic (optional)
> red pepper flakes (optional)
> salt to taste

Put black-eyed peas in medium saucepan; cover with water and cook until done (cooking time for fresh peas is a lot faster than for dried). Dried peas may also be soaked a few hours ahead to speed cooking and aid digestion.

Basil Mashed Potatoes

> 6–7 purple or golden Yukon potatoes
> 1 tbsp. butter (optional)
> 1/4 cup fresh basil, chopped
> 1 cup soy milk

While black-eyed peas are cooking, scrub and boil potatoes. When potatoes are done (tender enough for a fork to pierce through), drain liquid, add butter, chopped basil, and soy milk, and mash potatoes with a potato masher until ingredients are smoothly blended. Note: purple potatoes are very sweet and creamy—no butter needed to get a terrific, rich taste.

Spiced Beets and Greens

6–8 small or 4–6 medium to large beets
1/4 tsp. alllspice
1 clove garlic
2–3 leaves fresh sage (or 1/2 tsp. dried)
1 tbsp. olive oil
1 tsp. butter

While potatoes are boiling, remove and save stems and leaves from fresh beets. Scrub beets clean, removing any tough skin with a knife. Put beets into a medium saucepan, cover with water, add allspice, and bring to a boil. Reduce heat, cover with lid, and cook until fork tender (30 minutes or so). While beets are cooking, chop beet stems and greens into small pieces, and dice garlic. (If you are going to cook the okra recipe that follows this one, set beet greens aside and start preparation of the okra.) When the rest of the meal is done, quickly sauté greens, stems, garlic, and sage in 1 tbsp. olive oil until tender, stirring constantly for 3–4 minutes until done. Add salt to taste and 1 tsp. of butter for a richer flavor, if desired. Note: My thanks to Amadea Morningstar's *Ayurvedic Cooking for Westerners* for giving me the idea to cook beet greens this way.

Rosemary Okra

1 lb. fresh okra
2/3 cup cornmeal
1 tsp. freshly chopped rosemary (or 1/2 tsp. dried)
2 egg whites
light cooking oil (olive, canola, or sunflower are good choices)
salt and pepper to taste

If you're cooking the entire Southern Feast, start okra after you have black-eyed peas, potatoes, and beets going. Slice okra into 1/2-inch pieces and put into pastic bag. Add egg whites and coat okra, then add rosemary and cornmeal. Shake until pieces are thoroughly coated. Put 3 tbsps. oil into large skillet and heat on medium-high until oil is hot. Add okra mixture and stir, sautéeing for a few minutes until corn meal begins to brown. Reduce heat to low, cover and let okra steam itself, stirring occasionally, about 15 minutes, until done. Note: For okra lovers, this version uses a lot less oil than traditional frying. The rosemary gives it a new twist, and the okra has the same great taste and crunchy cornmeal coating, while keeping very moist and tender. The best of both worlds!

Summertime Squash

2 yellow squash and
2 zuccini squash, cut into bite-sized pieces
1 large or 2 small green onions, sliced
1/4 cup fresh oregano, finely chopped
(or 1 tsp. dried oregano leaves)
1 tbsp. olive oil
1 tsp. butter (optional)
salt and pepper to taste

Sauté all ingredients until vegetables are tender but not soggy. For variation, add 1/2 cup raw corn kernels as you cook, or 1/2 cup fresh green beans. A squirt of lemon juice stirred into the vegetables at the end of cooking is also very flavorful. Note: This recipe is great for vegetable gardener-cooks, because all of the ingredients usually ripen at the same time.

CALIFORNIA COOL

Wild Rice and Spinach Salad

1 cup uncooked wild rice, rinsed
4 cups fresh spinach leaves, chopped
2 sweet oranges (preferably seedless)
1 green onion (optional)
¼ cup pine nuts
salt to taste

Put rice in medium saucepan in 2 ½ cups water. Bring to a boil, reduce heat, and simmer with lid on until done, about 25 minutes. While rice is cooking, chop spinach leaves and put into medium bowl. Carefully cut peel off oranges, using a sharp knife and cutting off any white parts of the peel. Cut the membrane away from each orange section, allowing juice to drip into another small bowl as you cut; save juice for dressing. Mix orange segments, pine nuts, spinach, and cooled rice with:

Sesame-Soy Dressing

¼ cup toasted sesame oil
1 tbsp. lime or lemon juice
2 tbsps. Liquid Aminos (unfermented soy sauce)
¼ cup orange juice

Mix ingredients and serve over Wild Rice and Spinach Salad.

Tarragon Green Beans

      1 lb. green beans, cut or snapped into 1-inch pieces
      1/3 cup slivered almonds
      2 tsps. fresh tarragon or 1 tsp. dried
      1/8 tsp. mustard powder
      1/2 cup apple juice
      1 tsp. butter (optional)
      salt and pepper to taste

Toast almonds by cooking in small, dry skillet or saucepan on high heat for a few minutes, until almonds are a brownish color. In medium saucepan, combine all ingredients and barely cover with water. Bring to boil, cover with lid and simmer on high (rapid boil) until beans are tender (still bright green) but not soggy.

HAWAIIAN EXPRESS

Pineapple-Ginger Stir-Fry

1 cup fresh pineapple, cubed
1 cup carrots, thinly sliced
1 small can sliced water chestnuts
   (or jicama may be substituted instead)
1 medium sweet red pepper, cut into strips
1 clove garlic, minced
1 tbsp. red onion, finely chopped (optional)
1 tbsp. light cooking oil
2 tsps. grated ginger root
$1/2$ to 1 tsp. curry powder
$1/2$ cup unsweetened pineapple juice
1–2 tbsps. Liquid Aminos (unfermented soy sauce)
1 tbsp. flour (brown rice flour or corn starch may be substituted for
   wheat flour)
$1/3$ cup fresh cilantro, chopped
$1/3$ cup toasted sesame seeds
Cooked brown or white rice (optional)

If you are going to serve this meal with rice, start cooking it now, following package directions. Sauté garlic and onion in oil 1 minute, then add carrots and ginger and cook 3 more minutes. Add red pepper, water chestnuts, curry, and pineapple cubes and juice; cover and simmer on medium heat for a few minutes until red pepper is tender but not soggy. While dish is simmering, put Liquid Aminos, flour, and $1/4$ cup water into a small jar or container with secure lid, and shake until flour is dissolved. When red pepper is cooked, turn heat to low and slowly pour in flour mixture until the sauce forms to desired consistency. Toast sesame seeds in a small, dry skillet for 1 minute until seeds start to pop and turn brown; garnish dish with sesame seeds and cilantro leaves and serve over rice. Note: If you're trying to transition to lighter cooking but are still not to the vegetarian stage, toss in 2 uncooked chicken breasts, cubed, with the garlic and onion and cook as directed. Or add 8 ounces of cubed tofu as you add the carrots, for a more substantial meal.

Joyce's Apple Muffins

The following recipe (and variations) for muffins uses fruit, fruit juices and vegetables as well as a variety of flours and liquids. Ingredients may be changed to adapt to a particular mind-body type (barley flour and soy milk are good alternatives for Kapha). Switching to these muffins is a great way to reduce your feelings of dependence on yeasted bread without feeling deprived of baked goods. Once you get the hang of it, they take about five minutes to mix up, and about 15 minutes to bake.

Mix in a small sized bowl:
   2 egg whites or 1 whole egg or egg substitute
   1/3 cup oil (such as sesame, canola, sunflower or apricot oil)
   1/2 cup apple sauce and 1/2 cup plain apple juice
Mix in a medium sized bowl:
   1 cup oat flour
   1/2 cup oatmeal and 1/2 cup oat bran
   1 tsp. baking powder
   1/4–1/2 teaspoon cinnamon
   pinch salt (optional)

Grease and flour muffin pans. Blend wet ingredients into dry ingredients and spoon into muffin pans. Cook in a moderately low oven (300° F). 15 minutes or until done. Be careful not to bake too long or at too high a temperature, as muffins may dry out. Makes 12 muffins. Recipe may be cut in half.

For heartier Apple Muffins:
Blend in 1/2 grated red apple (with peel), 2 tbsps. raisins or nuts.

For Pumpkin Muffins:

Use ½ cup fresh cooked pumpkin instead of apple sauce, and add a few raisins, chopped figs, or dates (for sweetness), and a few nuts if desired. It's also possible to exchange the oat flour for barley, rye, or whole wheat flour, and use pumpkin pie spice instead of cinnamon.

For Banana Muffins:

Use 1 mashed banana instead of applesauce, and ½ cup rice milk instead of apple juice. Two cups brown rice flour may be used to replace oat flour, oat bran, and oatmeal.

For Blueberry Corn Muffins:

Use ½ cup fresh blueberries instead of applesauce, replace cinammon with allspice, and add a touch of grated lemon rind. Good with corn flour (which is finer than corn meal and requires a slower oven to keep muffins from drying out) or brown rice or rye flour.

Additional variations could include grated carrots to replace the pumpkin in the Pumpkin Muffin variation, or a few sun-dried tomatoes with grated zucchini, oregano, and basil for a savory flavor.

Note: It took me a while to get used to the idea of not eating yeasted bread, because bread was what I seemed to crave the most when stressed out (that was the Pitta in me, on chronic overload!). I have found that over the course of a year, my palate really shifted away from craving yeasted bread and sugary muffins as I introduced a variety of cooked grains into my diet: in hot breakfast cereals such as oatmeal, or millet cooked with almond butter (very tasty and hearty), and as side dishes or in casseroles, using grains such as quinoa, amaranth, barley, rice, and coarse corn meal for polenta. Cooking muffins using the recipe above helped me make the transition away from yeasted bread, and I have grown fond of all sorts of alternatives to bread such as tortillas, crackers, and flatbreads.

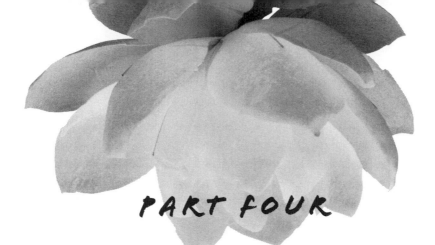

PART FOUR

Creating a Foundation
for Well-Being

What if time would bring joy
and life held meaning
and purpose
and self-love
What dreams do you dare to know . . .

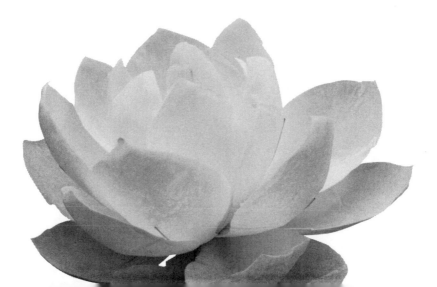

13

এ

Achieving Healthy Goals

Being clear on objectives is important in the process of achieving goals, but there are other factors that sometimes keeps us from achieving those goals while maintaining balance Ayurvedically. So often we rely on excessive willpower ("Pitta" energy) to reach our aims, which ultimately causes an imbalance such as burnout and medical problems, and perhaps a later inability to reach for those goals in the same way. In a more balanced approach, *how* the goal is met is as important as actually reaching the goal, and becoming more aware of the process of goal achievement helps to decrease frustration and stress. In Yoga class a student learns to hold a pose with effort and concentration rather than struggle and irritation. Like in Yoga, the more we understand our strengths and weaknesses, the more we are able to use this information to achieve our goals and maintain wellness and balance.

Seeking Balanced Goals

Sometimes accomplishing a goal is a mystery, because there are times when we don't know how we're going to succeed. In addition, some of us have grown up with unconscious tendencies to sabotage our success. Goal achievement is affected by our past and present environment, skills, and, most importantly, our belief systems. For example, often we know what we should do to keep ourselves healthy (eat well, exercise, find a balance between work and play, etc.) and yet time and again we fall short of where we want to be. Particularly with weight management, often our frustration about past failures and the feelings of emptiness that dieting conjures up keep us from looking at our situation more objectively, and harnessing our intellect to help us create lasting solutions.

In balancing, defining the goal is an important part of maintaining personal wellness—it is the first step in creating a foundation for a balanced and healthy goal-achievement process. In a modern world full of pressure to "keep up" and "fit in," we often fall short of choosing those actions that give us what we truly need. We unconsciously learn bad habits such as not paying attention to what our physical bodies and emotional psyches need or neglecting to build a foundation of personal beliefs that serves our health and wellness. In an age of recovery, where "self-help" books abound on gaining techniques for personal healing, we gobble up the info but may fail to integrate it; that is, we forget to give ourselves enough time to create a personal belief system, which allows our newly found habits and intentions to truly become a part of our lives.

It takes time to learn new habits. We need to have enough structure in our goal achievement to keep motivated and focused. From a more Ayurvedic point of view, identifying particular goals are better served by keeping in mind how each goal would nurture (or perhaps might cause imbalance to) our particular constitutions. In reality, there are times when we believe we have to put ourselves out of balance to gain a new skill or piece of knowledge that will help us maintain balance in the long run.

For example, I believed that by writing this book, I would be able to better achieve and maintain balance in my own life. But to be able to write this book, I had to change my approach to career, which meant a disruption in my finances while I gained the time, confidence, work habits, and ability to achieve my goal. I had to go through a period of transition that was often uncomfortable. I tried to minimize the disruption to my finances by saving enough money to give me a "cushion" before I changed my career, but I still had to deal with the anxiety that moving into the unknown causes. I knew that from time to time my doubts would cause me to feel worried and tense, causing the Vata aspect in me to manifest as stress. I also knew that my tendency to set aggressive goals and not allow enough time for rest and the creative process (thus inflaming my Pitta aspect) would be a factor. And lastly, I realized that working at home would increase the likelihood that my Kapha's natural desire for play would sidetrack my intentions.

So I had to plan a strategy to not only gain new skills, such as how to write a manuscript and prospectus for the publisher, for example; but also harness existing skills, like using my meditation and exercise practices as a way to manage increased stress. I had to remove obstacles, such as communicating to family and friends when I was available for them and when I needed my own time to think and write; as well as move into a part-time consulting status to keep myself financially solvent. I also had to create a new belief system, i.e., grow my confidence, to be motivated enough to do something I had never done before. This took interacting with others familiar with Yoga and Ayurveda, finding an agent to see if I could get published, considering the possibility of self-publishing and lecturing, experiencing the book as I wrote it to see if my beliefs and guidelines actually worked, and a myriad of other action steps and strategizing.

The only way I could accomplish such a complex task was to break the process down into simpler, more do-able steps. Knowing that too much stress would cause my imagination and writing ability to stop flowing easily and my concentration to scatter, I wrote down my goals. There were times when I couldn't see how I was going to finish, because of the imbalances that such a goal was invariably going to cause my constitution. This is where my belief in the logic of balancing my constitution Ayurvedically became useful, because I could always go back and restate my goal if my desire to write the book became a need that conflicted with my core values of getting enough rest, not overworking, and staying focused on the rewards that would come with accomplishing my goal.

My process of change helped me to understand how to change more consciously. I realized that the more I worked with my goals, the more I began to see how my past experiences and my environment helped or hindered my desire for well being and balance. I wrote my goals down and let them change as I began to grow and change. By being clearer about my goals, I was able to be more honest with my limitations and my needs. This process of understanding how to achieve a goal in a more balanced way cleared the way for my intellect to contribute to my evolution; it also allowed my heart to speak. The result was the improved ability to set a goal that identified what I truly needed as well as wanted.

One of my biggest breakthroughs in learning how to set and achieve healthy goals was in the area of weight management. My desire to learn more about Ayurveda and balance became very compatible with what I was learning about my emotional connections to food, and how my environment and past experiences influenced my ability to feel comfortable about my eating habits and self-image. As an adult, I was able to look back at my late teens and early twenties to the time when I had suffered greatly from an eating disorder and low self-esteem. I was able to acknowledge, bit by bit, my scars and bad habits, and see that using Ayurvedic concepts actually helped me to see new and more abundant choices. My fitness goals changed to include inner health, and I became kinder and more forgiving in my approach to accomplishment.

Table 7 is a weight-management planner that uses healthy goal achievement principles. The same process may also be applied to stress reduction and other personal growth goals you might have. Other processes that help in the achievement of balanced goals, such as quieting the mind through meditation or unleashing creative thought processes through guided imagining, are described in chapters 14 and 15.

The mind-body types (doshas) that primarily affect my constitution are:

_____ and _____

PHYSICAL

1. My weight management goal: _____

2. My eating patterns (cycles of hunger) when I am losing fat:

Morning _____

Midday _____

Afternoon _____

Evening _____

Late night _____

3. Exercise plan:_____

_____

4. Nurturing practices to calm hunger: _____

_____

MENTAL

1. What could disrupt my weight-management goals, and what can I do to make my goals a priority?

Work: _____

Table 7: Ayurvedic Weight Management Planner

People in my life: _____

Home environment: _____

Personal values: _____

Eating preferences/patterns: _____

Exercise: _____

Other: _____

2. What has kept me from reaching my weight-management goals in the past? How is my approach different from an Ayurvedic Balancing perspective?

_____

_____

3. Are my goals realistic? What goals can I set that I feel I can achieve?

_____

_____

4. How may I be fed mentally to support my weight-management goals?

_____

_____

EMOTIONAL

1. What emotional emptiness do I currently feel in my life?

_____

_____

2. What can I do to receive more love into my life and not be emotionally starved? What activities besides eating can I do to feel satisfied?

_____

_____

3. What are my basic needs to feel happy and well each day?

physical health	sense of well-being	good digestion
financial security	personal growth	organization/precision
beauty	managed hunger	stillness/peace
freedom	play/adventure	warmth/affection
other:		

SPIRITUAL

1. What am I grateful for each day?

_____

_____

2. What keeps me feeling connected to my sense of well-being and to others?

_____

_____

NEW BELIEFS

1. By developing new skills of self-nuturing, I am able to be fed on all levels so that physical hunger becomes a normal but not overwhelming aspect of life. What other new beliefs may I adopt?

_____

_____

_____

_____

14

ॐ

Engaging the Imagination

The seasons are an all-pervasive reminder of the natural cycle of change: as the seasons come and go, so we may grow awareness of a changing situation, embrace and appreciate newness, and let go of that which no longer serves. However, our emotional connections to self-image, past experiences, and the environment around us often make it hard to change our relationships to people, places, habits, beliefs, and things even when they have signaled a change. Emotionally letting go of loved ones or understanding that a daily habit or life pattern no longer serves our happiness is especially difficult when we forget that there are always new relationships, activities, and future pearls of wisdom to be found to further our evolution as human beings. Often change is seen as threatening and harmful, especially when early events in our formative years set a precedent for being fearful of change. Yet all of our awarenesses, gathered through interactions with other people and with our own internal feelings and thoughts, feed this growth and evolution. Just as the cycle of seasons occurs naturally, changes in our lives may serve the purpose of helping us gain awareness, hope, and a kinder, more flexible strength.

Dealing with Change

When trying to remove an obstacle that is keeping us from achieving a goal, it is often useful to write down exactly what the problem is, and also write down possible solutions that could be addressed if there were an abundant supply of resources and choices available. We dwell on what we can't do rather that focusing on what we can. Often we limit ourselves from seeing the choices available to us. We get stuck in old patterns through fear or skepticism or fatigue, which are respectively the Vata, Pitta, and Kapha aspects out of balance. Using our creativity and imaginations is the first step to uncovering new and perhaps better ways of solving old problems. Replacing your feelings of deprivation with possible choices can lead to the opening of new belief systems that support your desire for and achievement of balance and a healthy life.

Creative Problem-Solving—Playing the "What If" Game

1. What if you could identify one problem that you are currently experiencing regarding your well-being that you could begin to solve—what would that problem be?

_____

_____

_____

_____

2. What if you could change your current situation? How would that make you feel?

_____

_____

_____

_____

3. What if you could really visualize what you want to have happen? What would you want the outcome to be?

_____

_____

_____

_____

4. What if you had unlimited resources available to you to solve this problem in the most rewarding or constructive way? What resources, environments, skills would you acquire or change?

_____

_____

_____

_____

5. Now write down possible solutions, and break down into steps what it would take to implement those solutions. Don't settle for just any answer—look for several answers, and the one that truly satisfies you on all levels.

_____

_____

_____

_____

_____

Creating Tools for Change

When we begin to define balance we begin to develop an inner awareness of what our personal rhythms of balance are. Although each person's rhythms are different, we all seek to recognize and tend to the various types of hunger as they manifest in our bodies, thoughts, and feelings. Understanding hunger gives us the tools for change.

Here are some common hungers we face in our lives:

- Daily physiological hunger that prompts us to eat and sustain energy

- "Dis-ease" or illness caused by imbalances in our doshas or mind-body types

- Emotional hunger and the desire for love, joy, connection, and commitment

- Desire for personal growth that feeds our hunger of the spirit

These hungers give us specific daily needs:

- Physical movement/exercise to create strength, flexibility, and energy

- Clear thinking to achieve goals with realism, simplicity, and satisfaction

- Creative play/recreation to experience enjoyment and youthfulness

- Quiet time to calm, de-intensify, and release lethargy, heaviness, and stress

When we take the time to develop and use the tools for balance we may bring fundamental change to our mind-body constitutions:

- Vata moves from fear, nervousness, and restlessness to creativity, courage, faith, trust, calmness, and wisdom.

- Pitta moves from overintensity and unrealistic expectations to a softer focus that is more relaxed and less self-consuming.

- Kapha moves from a lack of motivation to the steady attainment of satisfying rewards.

Basic tools which allow us to actively create balance in our lives include:

- Ayurvedic cooking to balance hunger and provide physical and mental well-being.

- Regular physical exercise to consciously create energy

- Goal setting as a mechanism for self-inquiry to eliminate obstacles for growth

- Simple pleasures and nurturing practices to maintain happiness and joy

- Meditation and relaxation exercises to sustain equilibrium

As we decrease the resistance to change by understanding what we are truly hungering for, we see that consciously expanding choices creates abundance. If we seek to feed our hungers unconsciously, we often do so in a roundabout sort of way, often getting stuck on the obstacles to growth rather than focusing on developing the tools for change. Setting clear goals and visualizing the rewards of our efforts clear a path for creating positive habits that help support a lifelong foundation for well-being, while we shift away from what we "think" we should do to what we sense our bodies, minds, and feelings need for health. As we slow down our hurried worlds and introduce these basic tools for change step by step, we give ourselves time to make conscious choices. We learn new skills to enhance the capabilities of our mind-body constitutions. We gradually build a supportive environment through external interactions and internal beliefs that give us what we desire: personal balance.

15

Stress Reduction and Relaxation

I'm sure we've all heard the expression "a little stress is good for you." We all need motivation to push us past our fears, our hesitations, and our sluggishness. We all need skills to tolerate the stresses created by modern life, but more importantly, we need to understand which specific aspects of our lives create motivation and exhilaration, and which aspects push us past the point of comfort. As stress affects each of us differently, each of us has our own levels of tolerance to stress that affects our fitness levels and feelings of well-being. Stress is a relative concept—what may stimulate one person might exhaust another—and yet there are stresses in our society which we are all expected to master, such as taking personal responsibility for our emotional, financial, and physical well-being.

There are those on the other side of the spectrum who seem incapable of managing even basic levels of heightened expectation, ignoring everyone else's needs, and imposing their own habits, beliefs, and needs unconsciously on the rest of us. In an effort to find that middle ground between what we need and want and what others need and want, an important goal in managing personal stress is to become aware of what causes each of us stress, as well as being aware of how our actions might affect others. In other words, balancing stress becomes a daily intention of balancing our individual needs with the needs of those around us. When we begin to make conscious choices about what we want and need rather than unconsciously reacting to the people and environment around us, we greatly increase our ability to manage stress and find a balance between work, rest, and play.

The fact that stress is a subjective matter for each of us, however, is often ignored as we try to fit in to other people's patterns and meet expectations of job, family, and society. Let's look at the workplace as an example. If your goals and beliefs indicate one course of action, and your supervisor's or coworker's indicates another direction, increased stress is the potential result. If you desire a more conservative approach to a project, and your supervisor, teammate, or those you supervise are more reckless or driven to succeed "at all costs," you will feel the affects of increased tension mentally, emotionally, and physically as you work harder to satisfy someone else's objectives. Stress, therefore, may be defined as being torn between what we want to do and what we feel we should do. From an Ayurvedic perspective, stress may manifest as unfocused fearful Vata, overachieving Pitta, or undermotivated Kapha. It may also manifest as diseases, as alluded to in chapter 4. Often we try to achieve too much in a day, or achieve goals set for us by others rather than ourselves. We end up feeling stretched too thin, almost two places at once, putting a strain on our nervous systems, internal organs, and immunity to disease. Sometimes we shut down altogether, losing our ability to function and make clear choices about how we wish to spend our time. Regaining a sense of personal time and feeling like there is enough time to accomplish our goals is essential to stress reduction, and having clear goals helps us stay motivated, focused, and more evenly paced. It takes time, literally, to create our foundation; yet we often give away too much of our time to activities which do not truly nurture our well-being, and pay the price with emotional, mental, and physical strain.

Many aspects of our daily lives contribute to our stress levels, including life changes and personal growth, emotional fatigue from feeling deprived or "underfed," as well as uncertainty about the outcome of our actions and events around us. Overachievment or overwork takes its toll physically, as always thinking ahead to control the outcome of a task or endeavor may rob us of the pauses between the striving, and thus of a sense of enjoyment, satisfaction, and feeling of enriched living. Being uncertain about a future event or course of action, and worrying about it, also takes its toll. From a fitness perspective, striving to control our weight, dietary intake, and exercise habits can be exhausting if we are trying to use only control rather than a heightened desire for well-being combined with clear objectives and tangible rewards. Using the concept of balance, a middle ground between self-discipline and desirable, healthy goals can help to keep us motivated towards wellness. Once we understand what our particular mind-body types need to feel motivated and happy, it becomes easier to make healthy choices about how we spend our time, and recognizing the Ayurvedic traits of others gives us a greater awareness and understanding of what others expect or need from us.

1. What are some of the major stresses I feel in my life right now?

_____

_____

_____

_____

2. Would it be possible to spend more of my time nurturing myself, so that the balance of my time could be given more freely, without creating a sense of self-deprivation? (To see if your actual time spent in a week is congruent to the time you would like to spend, fill in the following list below.)

How much time do I spend each week on the following activities? In what areas do I need more time?

Career, vocation:

Sleep:

Family:

Exercise:

Friends, hobbies, and recreation:

Errands and chores:

Meditation and personal growth work:

Cooking and eating:

3. Having thus identified general areas in my life where I would like to spend more time on self-nurturing, here are three specific aspects of my life I would like to change, shifting them from an excess obligation, struggle, or unrealistic self-demand into positive goals that help reduce stress and increase feelings of well-being and balance:

1. _____

2. _____

3. _____

Reducing Stress

Regular "quiet" time creates an oasis of rest amidst the stressful pace of modern life. Having time to rest the mind leads to clearer thinking, and a greater ability to identify essential needs and desires, bringing balance and wellness into our lives. Taking a break from overstimulation (traffic, television, junk food, hectic work pace, etc.) puts less strain on our bodies and physical hunger; and because most of us have learned to comfort ourselves with food, we may reduce hunger by reducing situations which cause a buildup of stress (and the hunger for relaxation).

Having quiet time to meditate, enjoy personal solitude, rest, and let go of worries and expectations can, with practice, begin to positively affect how the "outside world" affects your inner peace. Whether it's finding time for simple pleasures such as reading the paper, taking a walk, or enjoying a meal—or developing more specific habits of contemplation, mindful exercise, and self-nurturing (including time for quiet sitting)—you can create preventative and restorative habits which help replenish those feelings of balance and well-being that the daily demands of modern life tend to erode. Below are three simple relaxation exercises you can do every day to contribute to your foundation of balance.

Quiet Sitting or Meditation

Sitting quietly is difficult for most Westerners, because we are impatient and unwilling to undergo the transition from restlessness, busy-ness, or boredom to receive the benefits of being still. Realizing that there are a myriad of teachers, styles, and objectives to choose from when considering meditation, a common objective of all meditation practices is to give yourself enough consistent time to become conscious of your true needs, and also to get beyond your thoughts to a place of relaxation and stillness.[15] Creating a meditation practice is a very personal process, and perhaps a challenging one for those trying to reduce stress. Here are some tips to actively include quiet time in your daily routine:

- Start by sitting quietly for ten minutes, eyes closed, in a place without distractions, preferably in the morning before you get "caught up" in your daily activities, or perhaps before your evening meal.

- Expand the sitting to twenty minutes, and if possible do this in the morning and evening. If you can't meditate in the morning, a break at lunchtime (like a walk or a "power nap") or before your evening meal would be beneficial. If you begin to meditate and fall asleep, chances are you needed the rest! If at all possible, resume your quiet sitting after your nap. It is also good to lie down after a meditation and absorb the quietness you have introduced into your thoughts and physiology.

- Some schools of thought suggest meditating before bedtime to quiet the mind before sleep. In any form, a regular meditation practice a few minutes a day is very beneficial. It helps to calm a busy mind, let go of worries or tensions accumulated during the day, soothe the body, and help you become accustomed to feeling quiet stillness throughout the day.

Guided Meditation (Reclining)

Lie flat on the floor or bed with hands at your sides and palms down. Close your eyes and focus for a few moments on your breathing, allowing your lungs and belly to slowly fill with air. Then release the breath, vocalizing out loud with an "ahhhhhh" sound if you wish. While breathing normally, visualize an opening in the top (crown) of your head, as if energy could freely flow inside this opening and through your body. Imagine this energy coming inside and relaxing all thoughts, muscles, ligaments, tendons, and organs. Guide this energy through your body three times:

First: through the crown of your head, down your ears, sides of your neck, shoulders, arms, and finally through your fingertips, relaxing each area as you focus on it;

Second: through the crown of your head, down your forehead and eyes, nose, mouth, chin, throat, heart, lungs, belly, groin, thighs, knees, feet, and finally through the toes, and;

Third: through the crown of your head, down the back of your head, along the base of your skull and neck, down your spine, the backs of your legs, and your heels.

Rest in this peaceful heaviness a few moments, inviting gravity to "let the floor hold you," moving slowly upright when done. This is a great way to begin the day before you get out of bed, and a restful way to end your day as you go to sleep. My thanks to Master Chen, professor of Chinese Soaring Crane Qigong, for teaching me this simple but effective exercise.

Self-Guided Imagining

Pick a goal that you would like to accomplish related to your fitness and well-being. After you have reached a peaceful place in your quiet sitting, or after you have finished the reclining meditation described above, focus on this goal and how it will feel to accomplish it and receive the rewards of your efforts. This affirming and motivating practice keeps you in touch with what your heart truly desires, and helps you develop the creativity to turn your desire into a reality.

Keeping the Peace

Bringing our daily lives back to a feeling of energized motivation rather than stressful accomplishment is a matter of choice—small choices we may consciously take each day which build one upon another like stepping stones, or unconscious choices which may or may not lead to sustained feelings of balance and equilibrium. As you begin to notice the various stresses in your life, you may be surprised at the amount of tension you unconsciously carry with you through the day. As we become more aware of stress, we may learn to:

- Identify specific stresses to be able to address them in a thoughtful and productive way.

- Use meditation techniques consistently, to allow the mind and body to relax. Meditation is beneficial for all mind-body types. If we choose, we may create enough time amidst the hustle and bustle of modern life to give ourselves enough rest and relaxation, so we may become aware of what we truly need to nurture our mind-body types.

- Engage in regular exercise to relieve built-up stress and give the body and the mind a chance to breathe. Exercising mindfully brings fitness to our physical bodies as well as to our minds and spirits.

- Become more aware of the variety of nurturing practices specific to our mind-body types that help maintain balance and equilibrium, and gradually introduce these new, healthier habits into daily life.

- Develop clear, healthy goals to reduce worry, increase focus, and create a rhythm of self-care.

As we become more practiced at making consciously nurturing choices, we become more unconsciously adept at living a life that offers less stress, healthier goals, and greater abundance. Ayurvedically reducing stress is not just a matter of avoiding those situations that cause us excess fatigue and worry; rather it's a process of gaining new skills to help us develop a stronger instinct for creating and maintaining health. It takes work to learn new skills, but we tend to make the process even more difficult by focusing on what feels like enormous change rather than understanding that change can happen in small, invited steps.

We've already discussed how having a comprehension of your personal constitution helps you understand your basic needs for health and well-being; more specifically, we've discussed how food choices and appetite are positively affected by an awareness of the impact of food on our physical and emotional well-being. We've also learned how engaging the imagination opens our minds to abundant choices, and in this chapter we've examined three simple exercises to begin to bring moments of relaxation regularly into your life. Chapter 16 discusses various physical exercises that help relieve stress, chapter 17 elaborates upon the notion of self-care, and chapter 18 uses the principles of healthy goal achievement to help you outline specific action steps you wish to take to create your own personal cornerstones of balance.

16

Balanced Exercise

As we have discussed in previous chapters, we may change the body's composition from fat-storing to fat-burning through a combination of exercise and conscious eating. Most people attempt to "diet," which often means limiting caloric intake to a point of actually lowering the body's metabolism and becoming less efficient at burning calories.

In a balanced weight-management program, the goal is to increase the body's capacity for fat-burning without creating an overwhelming physical and emotional sense of deprivation, while also paying attention to deeper hungers, which might negatively affect feelings of well-being and overstimulate appetite. If fat is burned moderately, the body will not create starvation signals that increase appetite to the point of overeating or eating for emotional comfort.

Eating excessive amounts of refined sugar may also affect the body's ability to convert sugar to usable rather than stored energy, as excessive levels of insulin (needed to metabolize excess sugar) may desensitize the body's ability to burn the sugar calories efficiently. Maintaining balance with the lean-to-fat ratio in mind is greatly aided by a combination of exercise, Ayurvedic eating that balances the appetite, relaxation exercises, and other forms of nurturing that calm the body and mind and provide an increased source of relaxed yet focused energy.

A balanced fitness routine includes three basic aspects: *musculoskeletal strength, cardiovascular capacity, and flexibility.* Often, participants at health clubs and gyms focus on developing muscle strength without flexibility or cardiovascular endurance, but that has begun to change with the introduction of a variety of classes, bikes, treadmills, and stair-stepping machines designed to get heart rates consistently elevated, and group exercise classes that teach various stretching exercises and even Hatha Yoga. It's unfortunate that there are still some "muscle-heads" who don't understand that making gains in muscle strength will be limited without a good stretching program, and that a healthy heart is just as important as bulging biceps. Many women will not introduce strength training into their workouts because they are afraid of "bulking up," and so miss the opportunity to increase bone density through weight-bearing exercise. What is particularly annoying is the way some Yoga instructors denounce weight training as adversely affecting mental and muscular flexibility, and cardiovascular exercise as an unconscious waste of time. The irony is that the fundamental aspects of strength, cardiovascular capacity, and flexibility are the same no matter what form of exercise you are doing, whether it's weight training, doing aerobics, or taking a Yoga class.

The basics of exercise are very compatible with the fundamentals of Ayurvedic Balancing. It's not that Yoga is better, although if done in a comprehensive way, performing Yoga postures increases muscular strength, flexibility, and cardiovascular capacity in addition to specifically focusing on more "internal" health of organs, tissues, and even mental and emotional well-being. Yoga has great appeal to emerging Westerners unsatisfied with their existing workout routine because Yoga is practiced in a mindful way; that is to say, the exercises are taught with the intention to get the student to focus on the specific muscles being used, the breath being generated, and the areas of tension that need releasing. Yet this is no different than a mindful weight trainer, who uses lung capacity and breath to increase performance during a lift, who focuses on the specific muscles being trained and how they are working and developing in relation to other muscles and to organs and connective tissue in the body, and who must actively stretch the muscles being worked so that strength gains are not diminished by tightness and soreness. There are gym-goers obsessed with thinness who do countless hours in "aerobics" classes or on cardiovascular machines; there are also those who incorporate cardiovascular exercise as part of a well-rounded routine, and who run and bike and dance aerobically because it gives them a sense of movement and enjoyment and accomplishment. A runner needs the same things as a Yoga student: lung capacity as well as limber yet strong muscles for good alignment and performance. Is running as mindful as Yoga? That all depends on the exerciser. A person can become obsessed with anything—even Yoga. An athlete works toward optimum performance, which means pushing past limits and becoming more in tune with what the body can and cannot do. A Yoga practice may also help us to confront our limitations and work with the body to develop greater breath and increased ability. Perhaps if we better understood the common principles inherent in any exercise, we would be more informed about the multiple benefits of a particular exercise and less likely to judge unfamiliar forms of exercise critically.

Each of us needs muscle strength and flexibility for good alignment of the spine and the ability to perform tasks (whether it's lifting the groceries or lifting a barbell). We all need cardiovascular activity to keep blood oxygenated, combined with healthy food to keep arteries clear and metabolism strong. All exercise may be done in a mindful way, paying attention to what we are asking our bodies to do, and why, and what effects these actions have on other muscles, organs, and our states of mind. And any exercise, even Yoga, can be overdone, or done incorrectly, setting the stage for injury and frustration. Personally, I have found that my competitive sports and weight training helped me to develop tremendous lung capacity, greatly aiding my Yoga practice which requires me to keep my breath flowing and use all of my lungs, not just breathing shallowly from the top third of my lungs. From sports, I developed a natural feel for the essential need to take long, deep breaths through the back of the throat to increase energy and therefore performance. Yoga, in turn, has taught me to breathe more evenly in daily life, becoming aware of how I hold my breath when tense or upset or fearful.

Yoga pointed to some of the imbalances in flexibility and strength my weight training and running had caused, and in turn my physical Yoga practice was greatly enhanced by my years of athletic training which gave me awareness and control of both muscles and breath. All exercise, not just Yoga, is enhanced by consistent effort; just as all fitness activities may feed a person on many levels if a mindful awareness is developed as to how the exercising is impacting other aspects of physical, mental, and emotional health. The principles of balance are not unique to Yoga postures, but more often than not they are taught more consciously than in other forms of exercise, and an awareness of these principles may help us develop a greater awareness of the inherent principles of balance, which can be found in other forms of fitness exercises.

Let's examine some of the fundamentals of strength, cardiovascular and flexibility training, noting their similarity to Ayurvedic and Yogic principles which form the backbone of balancing.

Strength Training

1. Strength training stimulates the body's metabolism on an essential level—glycogen storage—changing the mitochondria of the cells to a fat-burning rather than fat-storage mode. It also increases metabolism, which enhances the body's ability to utilize food for more immediate energy. (Yoga focuses on breathing, which oxygenates the blood and is the fundamental mechanism for the body to gain energy.)

2. If done correctly, weight training promotes balance between the chest, back, and legs by focusing on the strength of the trunk of the body. (Ayurveda asks us to know and understand our particular mind-body configurations, so we may actively take daily steps to nurture our constitutions and maintain personal balance.) Strength training also significantly helps maintain bone density as we age (just as understanding what we need Ayurvedically helps us maintain vitality and equilibrium, even as we go through personal challenges).

3. Train from the "core" of the body (the hip area) to the extremities, not vice versa. Like a tree, having a strong trunk gives better alignment and helps support the limbs. (Likewise, an Ayurvedic practice is built upon the awareness of what a person truly needs in relation to his or her specific mind-body configuration. Yoga focuses on developing the strength and flexibility of the spine, which is the backbone of movement and alignment. It also focuses on developing strength and flexibility of the mind, since our thoughts are the backbone of our actions.)

4. The three main muscle groups (chest, back, legs) should be trained with balance in mind, using weightlifting as well as stretching, since a muscle is only as strong as it is resiliant and flexible. When we only train what is easy, the weaker muscle group(s) become that much weaker in proportion to the stronger muscle(s). Often what we dread or avoid is what we need to train the most, creating doorways to balance. (Ayurveda and Yoga asks us to develop the awareness necessary to understand what we need, and then create a consistent practice to address those needs in a healthy, constructive way.)

5. You can build a muscle by developing the fast-twitch fibers through heavy lifting, and also by developing the slow-twitch fibers through higher reps with less weight. Muscle tissue is built by causing the body to lift a weight that is slightly heavier than what it is used to, thus creating small microtears in the tissues. As the body repairs these tears, it grows muscle and therefore strength. (In balancing, we learn to break down old beliefs and habits that no longer serve, to create a space for new ideas and greater, more conscious abundance.)

6. A sprinter has more fast-twitch fibers than a long-distance runner, whose emphasis is endurance rather than speed. As in life, when some days we "sprint ahead" and some days we "plod along"; combining the more explosive technique of heavy lifting with the more methodical technique of lighter lifting to help create a balanced physique. (In Ayurvedic Balancing, we come

to realize that some changes are more easily made than others, and that patience is one of the greatest tools we develop so that we may eventually gain the skill, through practice and consistency, to make positive, lasting changes.)

7. Intermediate and advanced weight trainers are best served by cycing their lifting days between "heavy" days (more weight, less reps) and "light" days (less weight, more reps). Lighter days give rest to joints, tendons, and ligaments while burning more calories, and heavier days give more rest time between sets and more shape to muscle bellies. (In Yoga class, some of the most significant gains in flexibility can come when a student is tired or physically "less than on top of their game." A student who is unable to rely on the Pitta quality of willpower to force changes usually by default allows the body to relax into the pose with less struggle—and thereby actually increases flexibility.)

8. In weight training, determining what areas need the most work helps you create a strategy to build up weaker body parts. (In Ayurveda, a student may more objectively see what his or her constitution truly needs, and therefore make more conscious choices which in turn nurtures well-being at deeper levels.)

9. Lifting weights can be similar to a Yoga practice when concentration and intention combine to create a series of moving poses interspersed with rest periods. Muscle growth (increase in strength) occurs if there is enough rest between workouts, just like a meditative frame of mind results when rest occurs between moments of effort (whether it be a weightlifting, a Yoga pose or daily life).

Cardiovascular Exercise

1. Any form of movement (walking, biking, jogging, swimming, dancing, etc.) that increases the heart rate to approximately 60–80 percent of the maximum heart rate over a period of not less than twenty and not more than

sixty minutes is considered aerobic and beneficial for burning fat. Anaerobic exercise such as weight training expands the heart's potential to do more work in short spurts and uses glycogen rather than fat as its primary fuel source. If you can carry on a conversation while you are exercising, without gasping for breath, you are probably in a fat-burning mode. In aerobic training, faster is not necessarily better; what helps is a moderate pace for a sustained period of time.

Likewise, in personal growth, some changes take time. If we are trying to shift our appetites from inflamed hunger to balance, we must address the imbalance(s) causing our hunger. Eating Ayurvedically greatly helps us to feel well nourished, which positively affects our state of mind and helps to ease feelings of emotional hunger and deprivation. Like cardiovascular exercise, Ayurveda looks for small, successive, and sustainable changes over time.

2. Often people who are running, biking, or taking aerobic class let their breath be a byproduct of their desire to move, rather than letting the breath be the focal point of the movement. Yoga focuses on consciously expanding the lungs and our ability to breathe. If we focus on exhaling thoroughly, the lungs will instinctively respond and try to fill themselves up. Eventually, Yogic breathing becomes a very natural response, positively affecting the breath in all forms of exercise as well as in stress reduction.

3. Cardiovascular exercise outdoors can give us recreation, which is a great stress release and source of enjoyment. As we have discussed previously, feeding ourselves on all levels is important in creating feelings of well-being and abundance, and those activities which allow us to "breathe" (both literally and metaphorically) help us to "lighten up" and let go of heavy thoughts. Introducing a variety of cardiovascular exercises into your routine helps you avoid overusing joints and muscles. If you find you are becoming emotionally dependant on certain forms of exercise—even Yoga—to give you a sense of well-being (rather like a "fix" than a consistent practice), you may be creating imbalance. Sometimes well-intentioned Yoga students

become too serious or ungrounded in their pursuit of spiritual growth; sometimes gym-goers take the "no pain, no gain" philosophy too literally. Unconscious growth usually means we grow in one area (while causing an imbalance in another), but as we become more aware of our actions and their repercussions, we begin to make more inclusive choices which positively affects our life. In cardiovascular exercise, a healthy heart is the focus; in Yoga, breath is life.

Flexibility

1. Performing Hatha Yoga postures regularly helps give the body flexibility and balanced strength, increases breath, and teaches concentration through a relaxed focus. Each pose affects the body differently, and poses may be used to nurture particular mind-body types. There are many different styles of Yoga that appeal to different needs and interests: some schools emphasize holding poses for several minutes at a time, using props such as straps and pillows to help the body ease into a pose; others are more athletic and implement the use of more vigorous poses in a posture "flow" or sequence; yet other classes vary their focus from class to class and teach a combination of vigorous and gentle poses.

2. Certification programs for Yoga teachers are still very inconsistent from studio to studio, so it's up to the student to find quality instruction. Some instructors focus on the more nurturing aspects of the poses, with emphasis on emotional and spiritual growth. In contrast, some schools are almost militaristic, teaching strict form or relying on specific, vigorous routines that are taught in repetition. There are some studios that use the "warm room" technique, sometimes getting the temperature of the room to well over 100 degrees (to aid in the body's ability to release physical tension, and to help the mind develop focus and intensity). If you are a Pitta-type person, you may be drawn to these intense forms of Yoga, which might actually cause more imbalance because of the intense heat and reliance on willpower. Exposure to different forms of Yoga is therefore beneficial if

you're a beginner, so you may make a more informed choice as to which type of class is right for you. Often our Yoga needs change with our lives; sometimes a vigorous class is what you need to help you work through obstacles; sometimes a more nurturing approach to heal an injury or emotional wound. The best judge of your needs, ultimately, is you.

3. Do some stretching and warm-up before you start any exercise, and five to ten minutes of stretching after you exercise. This way, you avoid muscle pull and injury before you start, and also reap maximum stretching benefits at the end of your workout, when your body is warmed up and probably more relaxed from the physical exertion. If possible, try to hold stretches for at least one to two minutes. If you can't hold a stretch that long, you may be trying to force the stretch to a place of extreme discomfort. On a scale of one to ten, with ten being the hardest, try for a place in the stretch that feels like a six or seven so that the discomfort is manageable.

4. Use your breath to create greater flexibility. Breathe in as deeply as possible, to create enough energy to work the muscle during the stretch, and increase the position of the stretch as you exhale, creating a rhythm of breathing in as you hold the stretch, and breathing out as you deepen the stretch a bit further. Use small adjustments and increments when deepening the stretch. Sometimes the stretch occurs in your head, as your thoughts get used to the idea of eventually being able to loosen up a tight place. The body will eventually follow the mind, and allow the physical stretch to come when ready.

Notice if you are asking your body to stretch, or demanding the muscles to loosen up. Be kind to yourself, but firm (and don't overstretch); those muscles really want to loosen up, even if they protest in the process!

Health Clubs

There are many factors to consider when joining a health club, obvious ones being cost and proximity to where you live or work. Does the club or gym have a variety of classes and programs to keep pace with your chang-ing needs over time? What kind of instruction do they give you, and are the instructors degreed or certified by a nationally recognized certification pro-gram? Is there adequate space for stretching, and places to relax your mind and body as well as get motivated?

Health clubs, workout studios, and gyms provide you with incentive to exercise, even on those days when you could easily drive straight home after work and aim for the couch. Knowing that friends will be there, getting into a healthy routine (which your body begins to ask for over time), having an enjoyable place to let go of tension and recreate—all are benefits that fitness facilities can give. It's important to be honest with yourself and admit if a particular club, studio, or gym does not feel right for you; in other words, just because you think you should do something doesn't mean you will, par-ticularly if the routine or facility doesn't feel comfortable or rewarding over time. There is always a period of discomfort or unsettledness when begin-ning any new habit, but you also have an instinct that will tell you if the fit-ness routine or location is something you can maintain over time. As with most choices we make in life, give yourself enough time to experience the newness, and also give yourself permission to change if the program or facil-ity is no longer right for you. The important thing is to keep exercising, keep exploring new options when appropriate, and remember that enjoyment is a great motivator to keep fitness as a regular part of your lifestyle.

Creating a Workout Program

There are lots of variables to consider when creating a workout routine: what your goals are, how much time you have, what you enjoy doing (versus what you feel you need to do, which affects motivation), the facilities and instruc-tion you have available to you, and your current physical condition. Getting at least thirty minutes of exercise three times a week is a good start. I have found that I have gone through different phases in my life, even though I was still addressing the three basics of exercise (strength, cardiovascular conditioning, and flexibility). In my younger days I was a competitive athlete focusing on cardiovascular exercise such as basketball and running; then I shifted to body-building (while maintaining some cardio and stretching); and then to Hatha Yoga as the predominant exercise form. Now I do all three, finding that a couple of times in the gym lifting weights helps release the Pitta intensity; whereas a few Yoga classes soothe jumpy Vatta and the bike riding or hiking allows my Kapha aspect to recreate and play. Whatever form or forms of exercise you choose, remember to get the three basics in, for strong yet flexible muscles and a healthy heart.

According to Deepak Chopra's *Perfect Health,* different body types are nurtured by different exercises.[16] People with a lot of Vata in their constitutions do well with exercises that allow them to have bursts of energy without tiring too quickly. Yoga and aerobics classes are beneficial, as well as walking, short hikes, and light bicycling. From a fitness point of view, Vata types are not particularly drawn to lifting weights as it can seem too strenuous, even though their frailty would be served by weight-bearing exercise for bone density and strength. If even a short weight-training session doesn't appeal, certain Yoga poses may help build strength and cardiovascular capacity. Class settings are good for Vatas, who benefit from the camaraderie of classmates and the focused instruction of a teacher who can prevent Vata types from overdoing and exceeding limits.

Pitta-type exercisers like challenges and have moderate endurance. Skiing, brisk walking, jogging, hiking, and swimming are all good exercises, but Pitta-influenced people have to be careful of getting overly competitive because of their fighting spirit. Often Pittas will force themselves to exercise but not find pleasure in their efforts, even though they like having a sense of accomplishment. Exercises that soothe and release intensity are very nurturing for Pitta; more aggressive pursuits like weight lifting are enhanced if performed with a more mindful, meditative approach.

Kapha-type people are best equipped for moderately heavy exercise, and weight training, running, aerobics class, and rowing are good for maintaining lean muscle mass while burning fat. Kaphas are endurance oriented and increase sports performance when they include flexibility and balance training. Breaking a good sweat feels good to Kapha, helping them release excess fat and water.

Chopra reminds us that Yoga offers poses good for all three mind-body types, much like Amadea Morningstar's *Ayurvedic Cooking for Westerners* offers nutritious and tasty meals that appeal to all constitutions. His book, and others which are listed in the bibliography section of this book, are excellent sources of Yoga routines that are designed to Ayurvedically nurture the body, mind and spirit. There are also some Yoga poses to increase back strength and flexibility in Table 8. A book, however, is no substitute for hands-on instruction in a class setting. Not only do you benefit from seeing other, more practiced students doing the poses, but you get specific corrections and pointers pertinent to you, not to mention the support from students who, like you, are furthering their growth and ability by the pursuit of Yoga. In the best of both worlds, you may begin to develop the ability to listen to what your particular constitution needs, while benefitting from instruction and fellowship, striking a balance between being a student and becoming your own teacher.

In summary, the goals for a balanced exercise program are:

- To develop a strong yet flexible core, focusing on lower back and abdominal health

- To use breath to energize the body consciously, paying attention to the dialogue between mind and body

- To combine exercises effectively to create balance, not imbalance

Table 8 demonstrates basic warm-up stretches, abdominal and lower back training, weight training basics and suggestions for Yoga poses.

Table 8: Balanced Exercise Routine

A. *Warm-Up Stretches*

If you are about to start an exercise routine, take the time to oxygenate your blood and expand your lungs with deep breaths. Give yourself time to take in five deep breaths, counting five seconds to inhale, and five seconds to exhale. It only takes a minute, and if done throughout the day, it helps keeps tension from constricting both lungs and thoughts.

1. Neck and upper spine

Tuck your chin in as far as you can, lowering it onto the breast bone if possible. You should feel a stretch all the way down your spine to your waist. Hold this position for at least ten counts and breathe normally. Slowly look to the right, reaching your chin as if it could rest on your right shoulder, and hold it for ten counts; then slowly look to the left and do the same. Finally, allow the head to fall back, being careful not to pinch the back of the neck.

2. Shoulders

Pretend there is a dot painted on the sides of your shoulders, and draw a circle with those dots by rolling your shoulders up, back, down, and forward—keeping the neck relaxed as you do. Draw five circles in this direction, and then repeat in reverse so that your shoulder rolls start toward the front. Next, stand with feet hip-width apart. Holding a five-pound weight in the right hand, and keeping the right elbow and upper arm "glued" to your body, swing your weighted hand out to the side, and back, as if your upper arm and elbow were a door jamb and your forearm and weighted hand were the door opening and closing. Remember to keep your shoulders back, your chest out, and your elbow "attached" to your rib cage, even if it means you won't be able to swing your arm open as much. This exercise is a good indicator of tightness in the shoulder area; if done consistently, the shoulder will start to open up and help prevent injury.

Lastly, stand with feet hip-width apart. Holding a five-pound weight in the right hand, move the right hand in a circle in front of the body, as if the weighted hand were the minute hand of a clock circling around the clock's face. Do ten complete circles with the right hand, then hold the weight with the left hand and complete ten circles.

3. Chest

Clasp your hands together behind your back and roll the shoulders back and down. If you are near an open door, stand in front of the door opening, raise your left arm at your side so that your elbow makes a 45-degree angle (like an L) and place the elbow and hand on the door jamb, leaning into your shoulder until you feel a stretch. Then repeat this for the right arm. To further open up the chest and shoulders, stand in front of a sturdy pole, and grab onto the pole by reaching behind you with your hands. Firmly gripping the pole with both hands, and positioning the feet near the base of the pole, lean away from the pole, suspending your body away from the pole and sticking your chest out as if you were a mermaid on the bow of a sailing ship. Really extend the shoulders back, feeling an opening in both chest and shoulders.

4. Torso/Hips

Our spines are meant to move in all directions—side to side as well as forward and backward. With your feet shoulder-width apart, stand tall and raise your arms overhead, reaching up first with the right hand, and then the left, imagining that your fingertips can actually touch the ceiling if you reach far enough. Get on your tiptoes as you reach, and feel the stretch open up the hip and torso area. Then with hands placed on the back of your hips and your legs and seat tightened to support the lower back, allow the chin to reach toward the ceiling, the neck to become long (not pinched) and the shoulders to roll back, allowing the chest to open. Finally, bend at the waist and allow your arms to reach toward the floor. Touch your shins, or if possible, the floor, with your hands and hold for a minute. For added stretch in the hips, lean into the left hip (lifting up the right heel if you need to) and count to ten, and then lean into the right hip (lifting up the left heel if necessary) for ten counts. Repeat this process until you've held the stretch for at least sixty seconds. If you stand in place or sit a lot, try to release the lower back every hour or so.

5. Quadriceps

To stretch the quadriceps muscles out, stand tall with feet together and put your weight on the right foot. Then bend the left leg behind you at the knee until you can hold your left foot in your left hand. Keep your knees as close together as possible, balancing on the right foot for ten-to-thirty seconds until you feel a good stretch in the front of the leg. Repeat the stretch, this time balancing on the left foot and stretching out the right thigh.

6. Calves and hamstrings

Bend forward at the waist until your hands are touching the ground, bending the knees if you need to. Be careful to protect your lower back. Walk the hands out about three to four feet in front of you, and then straighten one leg, leaning into that heel and holding for ten counts, and then the other leg. If possible, put both heels on the ground and hold for up to sixty seconds. An alternative version to stretch the calves is to face a wall, place your palms against the wall, fingertips up, and push the left heel back until the leg is straight and the heel is flat on the floor. If you don't feel a stretch in the calf muscle, move the foot back until you do. Then stretch the right leg.

B. Abdominal and Lower Back Care

I've found that a fundamental principle of weightlifting applies to abdominals too, namely, it's not so much how much time you spend, but rather the intensity of the exercise that counts. Just doing lots of abdominal crunches is often not enough, because the muscles of the lower back and neck can become sore as form breaks down from fatigue. Also, as a particular muscle becomes used to a specific amount of work, it requires an increase in the intensity (or difficulty) of the exercise to maintain peak performance. I suggest you spend five to ten minutes or so doing a lower-back abdominal routine after your initial warm-up stretches, to strengthen your core and prevent injury.

You can easily fit the routine in anywhere (gym, home, hotel room) so that your abs and lower back get exercised on a regular basis.

To increase flexibility and strength, I recommend you do this routine four to five times a week; to maintain, do the routine three or four times a week. I've included warm-up exercises before the abdominal work as well as stretching exercises afterward, so that your lower back (which is part of your body's "core" of strength) gets included, too.

Begin by loosening the lower back, hamstring, and groin:

1. Hip and Hamstring Opener

In a standing position, with feet hip-width apart, gently bend forward and reach for your toes. If your hands cannot touch the floor, rest them on your shins. Relax your neck, letting your eyes gaze at your shins. Lean into the right hip, allowing the left leg to bend and the left heel to lift up. Breath deeply and hold this position for ten counts, allowing the exhale of breath to help you release tightness in the right hip. Then switch sides and lean in to the left hip, noticing if you are tighter on one side of your body (which is typical, since most of us are not ambidextrious but favor one side over the other). Also take into account previous neck and back injuries when performing this or any exercise, being aware of the difference between pain (the stiffness from tight muscles trying to loosen up) and injury.

2. Straddle Stretch

In a seated position on the floor, open the legs to a straddle position. Lift the arms overhead, gently twist your body to the left, and lean your chest over the left leg, holding onto your shin (or left foot, if possible) and breathing for ten counts. Do not bounce; rather, try to increase the stretch by taking in a deep inhale, and then bringing your nose closer to your left foot on the exhale. Ideally, a deep stretch should be held for at least sixty seconds, depending on your existing flexibility. See if you can work up to a longer period of stretch, without straining or creating excess pain. In other words, on a scale of one to ten, try to hold the stretch at the intensity of level seven (enough effort to make progress but not an excess amount which causes you to tighten up and struggle). Then change legs, noticing if one leg is tighter than the other. If one side is significantly tighter, you may want to hold the tighter side for a longer period of time, until your body develops a more symmetrical flexibility.

3. Knee to Chest

Lying flat on your back with legs extended, bend the right knee and bring the right leg up toward the chest. Clasping the knee two inches below the kneecap, pull the knee to your chest, while keeping your back on the floor as well as your left leg on the floor. Keep your chin tucked and your gaze toward your bellybutton. You may need to flex the toes of the left foot toward you to keep the left leg from lifting up off the ground. As you bring your right thigh toward your chest, keep your shoulder blades touching the ground and your elbows in toward your torso. You may need to move the right knee toward your side, to continue the stretch and release the groin muscle. Repeat on the other side. Then, bend both knees toward you and wrap your arms around your knees, grasping at opposite elbows if possible. Keeping your back flat and your chin tucked, press both knees together and press your lower back into the floor. Hold each position for at least thirty seconds.

Now focus on strengthening the abdomen.

Even though the abdominal wall is one muscle, there are different "sections" of that muscle you can isolate, for increased strength and intensity of exercise. There are two basic premises to this collection of exercises. The first is that you start out at the beginning level, until you are sure that you have isolated the abdominal muscles properly and can perform each level of the exercises in good form. This is very important for avoiding injury to the neck and lower back. The second premise is that you are eventually going to increase intensity in two ways: by reducing the resting time between sets, and by increasing the difficulty of the exercise. Because your abdominals have the most strength in the beginning of the routine, we start with a more difficult exercise first, to maximize the amount of work your abdominals can do. There are a total of five exercises to this basic abdominal strengthening.

4. Crossovers

Begin by lying flat on your back, hands tucked under your head. Bring the left knee to the right elbow in a gentle twisting motion, then let left leg rest and upper body come back to a fully reclining position, where the floor is completely supporting the weight of your body. (In other words, allow the abdominal muscle to completely disengage from supporting your leg.) Then bring the right knee to the left elbow, and disengage. Do this for twenty times, each leg. Make sure you bring your knee to your elbow, instead of your elbow to your knee, so that you aren't pulling with your shoulders or neck but rather using just your abdominal muscles.

Beginning level: rest your feet and head on the ground between each "twist" of knee to elbow, for twenty counts each side.

Intermediate level: do twenty repetitions each side continuously, without pausing to rest the abdominal muscles.

Advanced: do twenty repetitions each side, with feet and head gliding along the floor, instead of resting between each twist. Be careful to build up your strength gradually, so that you are not compensating with shoulders, neck, or lower back, but rather using only the strength of the abdominals. Focus on keeping your abdominal muscles tight, as if you were driving your bellybutton through your spine and into the floor. Eventually you should be able to crisscross your legs back and forth smoothly, as if you were riding a bicycle.

5. V Crunches

Lying flat on the floor, with arms by your sides and legs together, simultaneously bring your chest and your knees toward each other so that your thighs and your chest form a V shape. Be very careful to pull with your abdominal muscles and not with your chin or neck. After each crunch, bring your head and feet back down to rest on the floor.

Beginning level: Twenty repetitions, with rest in between each crunch.

Intermediate level: Twenty repetitions, with no rest in between each "crunch" (but being careful to come back to the starting position, so the abs get a good stretch between each crunch).

Advanced level: Twenty repetitions with no rest, and with feet and upper body gliding back and forth in a continuous, smooth movement without resting on the floor between crunches.

6. Regular Crunches

Lie on your back with knees together, and bend your knees so that your feet rest on the floor, close to your buttocks. With hands lightly clasping your head, raise the chest up until you feel a contraction of your abdominal muscles. Hold it for a second or two, and then slowly release back down. As you contract your abs, try to press your belly-button down through the spine and into the floor (creating a flat back position each time you crunch). Do not raise up with your chin or neck first, as this causes strain and utilizes more shoulder muscle than abdominal muscle. It's not important that your chest raises a lot; what is important is to contract the abdominals as much as you can.

Beginning level: Twenty repetitions, with your upper body resting on the floor between each crunch.

Intermediate level: Twenty repetitions with no pauses between repetitions, holding the crunch for a count of three.

Advanced level: Bring your feet in as close to your buttocks as possible, and keep knees together during all phases of the crunch. If possible, squeeze buttocks together as your chest in raising up, pushing your tailbone up slightly. (You will feel the contraction a bit lower down the abdominal wall this way.)

7. "Feetless" Crunches

Instead of keeping your feet on the ground, keep them up so that your shins are parallel with the ground. Be careful to push your bellybutton down through your spine to the floor, to keep the back from arching.

Beginning level: do ten reps continuously.

Intermediate level: add another ten reps, only this time your legs are straight and lifted so that your legs and torso form a right angle. Keep your legs straight and knees together, lifting your chest up and down while holding the legs upright and still.

Advanced level: as you lift your chest up on the last ten reps, try to lift your toes into the air. This means that you are going to try to lift from your tailbone, so that your legs remain in the air but lift slightly from the hips. You will feel this contraction low in the abdominal wall.

8. Rope Pull

In a seated position on the ground, bring feet toward buttocks with knees together. Lift your right arm up as if you were pulling yourself up on a rope, and then raise the left arm as you lower the right arm. Keep your abdominal muscles contracted, with your bellybutton pressed toward your spine. Do this for ten reps.

Beginning level: ten reps, with enough space between the feet and buttocks to create a 45-degree angle between the back of the knees and your calves/hamstrings.

Intermediate level: bring feet in closer to the buttocks, for ten reps.

Advanced level: lower your torso down, rep by rep, as if you were really lowering your torso with an imaginary rope. To make it even more difficult, you can "lower" your torso down slowly for the first five repetitions, and then lift it slowly for the last five repetitions.

Remember—use your abdominal strength, not your lower back. Don't forget to stretch the abdominal wall out after you have done your crunches.

This way your abs will have strength and suppleness, which helps to keep you injury-free.

9. Cobra Stretch

After finishing your abdominal exercises, lie on your chest and stomach with your legs fully extended and feet touching. Place your hands on the ground so that they are resting under your chest. Slowly push up with the arms, getting a good stretch in the abdominal muscles. Be careful not to raise up too high and create a pinching feeling in your lower back. To support your lower back, keep your buttock muscles tight, and press the tops of your feet firmly into the ground. This stretch should feel good; if you feel pain in the lower back and shoulders, lower the chest closer to the floor so that only the abdominals are getting a good stretch.

10. Puppy Stretch

Sitting on your feet and knees "Japanese style," slide your hands forward so that your forehead is resting on the floor and your hands are stretched out on the floor in front of you. This should give you a nice release in your lower back, as well as stretch out your shoulders. Breathe deeply, trying to breathe from the backs of your lungs (rather than shallowly with the upper part of the lungs). Hold this position for at least thirty seconds, to enjoy the benefits of the relaxation it brings to your body.

11. Cat Stretch

Resting on your hands and knees, lift the chin up and rest the back of the head gently on the neck, while simultaneously extending the chest out and arching the back. We've seen cats do this all the time, right after they get up from a nap. After arching the chest, drop the head down and bring the chin to the chest, while pushing the spine up through the hands to form a rainbow with the torso. This backward and forward movement of the spine, done slowly and gently, helps to loosen up the lower back and relieve tension. Remember to inhale as you look up, and exhale as you drop your chin.

C. Basic Weight Training

The basic weight-training exercises for the three main muscle groups are:

Chest: Primary movement—press (barbell, dumbbell, or exercise machine)

Secondary movement—fly (dumbbell, cable, or exercise machine)

Back: Primary movement—row (barbell, dumbbell, cable, or exercise machine)

Secondary movement—cable pulldowns and pullovers (with dumbbells or machines)

Legs: Primary movement—leg press, squat, lunge

Secondary movement—extensions, leg curls

Remember, training these "core" muscle groups stimulates the more peripheral muscles such as arms and shoulders. Conversely, training arms and shoulders for a more muscular look, without doing the basics for chest, back, and legs, will eventually lead to plateaus in strength gains (and more importantly, potential injuries from the imbalance created). Primary movements build strength, while secondary movements supplement the primary movements and also help shape the muscle.

Additional exercises include:

Arms: Bicep curls (dumbbells, barbells, cables, and machines)

Tricep "dips" and pushdowns (cables and machines)

Shoulders: Primary movement—overhead presses

Secondary movement—lateral arm raises

Abs: Crunches and leg lifts

Beginning weightlifters are best served with sets of ten reps, combining the concepts of heavy and light lifting. For more experienced lifters, cycle "heavy" days of doing six-to-eight reps per set until you progressively reach your maximum weight (called "pyramiding" an exercise) with lighter days where you do ten-to-twelve reps per set with 20 to 25 percent less weight.

A *beginning* routine may include three-to-five sets of ten reps, two or three times a week:

Chest: Dumbbell press and dumbbell fly on a flat bench, or exercise machines

Back: Dumbbell or cable rows and a cable pulldown

Legs: Machine presses or lunges, plus leg curls and extensions if desired and two-to-three sets of ten reps per minor body part, performed two-to-three times a week.

A more advanced routine would increase the sets to seven-to-ten sets per body part, dividing the total exercises over a two-or-three-day period and cycling from heavy to light periods. Also, in more advanced routines, changing the angle of the bench to incline or decline affects the area of emphasis and adds difficulty to the pose. Remember, strength training is progressive: as the body becomes accustomed to lifting a particular weight or performing a particular exercise, you must introduce more weight or increase the difficulty of the exercise to maintain and increase strength.

Note: If you would like to combine cardiovascular exercise such as bike riding or group exercise class with strength training, I suggest you perform the strength training exercises (which burn primarily glycogen) first, so that more fat stores are burned during the cardio portion of the workout.

D. Yoga for Strength and Flexibility

After doing the warm-up stretches and abdominal-lower back routine, I usually choose to do either a series of Hatha Yoga postures or a series of weight training exercises. Whatever form of exercise you choose, make sure your focus emphasizes lower back strength and conscious breathing. As Yoga teacher Richard Miller reminds us: "So many students have low back pain, and strengthening is the way to overcome the low back difficulties. If forward bending is given too much, too soon, back pain will either develop or will not go away."[17] Miller therefore emphasizes strengthening the back in the beginning, middle, and ending of a Yoga routine. He also suggests that breathing should be synchronized into every movement of the pose, from beginning to end, as there are greater benefits to the body's immune system when exercise is performed with conscious breathing. Here are some basic poses that will help you develop strength and flexibility. I strongly recommend that you learn these poses first in a class setting with an experienced teacher, to avoid any injury.

1. Pranayama (Breathing)

Take a few moments to oxygenate the lungs. Stand tall with feet together. Interlock the fingers and lift the arms up so that your chin is resting on your knuckles. As you begin a deep inhale for five counts, lift the elbows up past the top of your ears, while pressing your chin into your knuckles. Now tighten your buttocks, gently lean the head back over the nape of your neck, and exhale for five counts, drawing your elbows together in front of your face. In effect, your arms are serving as a giant bellows, first helping to draw air into the lungs as you inhale, and then helping you squeeze the air out of your lungs as the elbows come together. Repeat this pose five times, and then stand for a few moments with arms at your sides and palms facing outward. This resting position is called Mountain Pose.

2. Half Moon Pose

Stand tall in Mountain Pose, with feet together and arms at your sides. On inhalation, lift your arms out from the sides of your body, palms facing up. Continue to lift your arms until they reach over your head, and your palms meet. Pressing your palms together, with one thumb crossed over the other to keep the hands in place, tighten your buttocks, stretch tall, straighten your elbows and exhale as you reach your torso and hands to the left. Your objective is not to crunch over on your left hip or bend forward at the waist but rather reach up with your arms and hands so that the movement of the spine is upward and then to the side. Keep the throat relaxed, lift up from the back of the spine while your torso is bent, and make a subtle crescent shape with the right side of your body, breathing normally for five counts. If you feel a pinch in your lower back, you have bent too far to the side. Gently release back to center, palms still pressed together over your head, and repeat to the right. Then come back to Mountain Pose and take in a few more breaths.

3. Lunge

Standing tall, position feet so they are hip-width apart. Breathe in, and on an exhale bend your knees and bend forward at the waist, walking the hands down the legs until they reach the floor. Be very mindful of any lower back stiffness or previous injury. Keep your head down and relax your neck. Then inhale, stretch your right leg directly behind you, rest your weight on the ball of your foot (with toes curled), and gently drop the right knee to the floor as you lift your head and gaze straight ahead. Hold this position for at least five counts while breathing normally, and then carefully bring your right foot forward so that it is resting next to your left foot, hip-width apart. Repeat for the left side, extending the left leg back, and then moving your left foot back to center next to your right foot.

Instead of coming back to an upright position, transition into Downward Dog.

4. Downward Dog

Bent at the waist and your feet hip-width apart, walk your hands out in front of you on the floor until your body is forming an upside-down "V," with hips lifted and feet and hands fully pressed into the floor. Relax the head and neck, feel the stretch in the backs of your calves, the lower back and the shoulders and hold for at least five counts while taking in full, deep breaths.

Instead of coming back to a standing position, transition to Cat Pose.

5. Cat Pose

While still in Downward Dog, bend your knees until you are resting hands and knees on the floor, like a cat. Inhale, lift the chin up and rest the back of the head gently on the neck, while simultaneously extending the chest out and arching the back. Then on exhalation, drop the head down and tuck the chin in to the chest, while pushing the spine up through the hands to form a rainbow with the torso. Do this forward and backward movement three times, paying special attention to the breath.

Instead of coming back to a standing position, transition to Half Locust Pose.

6. Half Locust

Lie belly-down on the floor with hands at your sides and legs completely extended, feet touching, head resting on your chin. One arm at a time, slide your hands under your thighs, palms facing the floor, so that your body is resting on your hands. Take a deep breath, exhale, and on an inhale lift the right foot up (so that the ball of the right foot is reaching for the ceiling), while simultaneously keeping the buttocks contracted and the right leg straight. The left leg remains passive and resting on the left hand. Breathe deeply and hold the right leg up for five counts. Be careful not to pinch the lower back—it is not important how high the right leg is lifted, but rather that the buttocks are contracted while the leg is being lifted. On exhalation, slowly lower the right leg, and then repeat with the left leg. Stay on the floor and transition to Seated Head to Knee Pose.

7. Seated Head to Knee Pose

Sit on the floor in a straddle position, with torso upright and legs extended to form a "W." Keeping the right leg extended, bend the left knee and move the left foot so that the ball of the left foot rests against the inside of the right leg, just above or at the knee. Bending the right leg if necessary, grasp the ball of the right foot with the hands, interlocking the fingers under the foot so that the ball of the foot rests in your interlocked hands and your thumbs rest on the top of the foot. Inhale, and on an exhale, slowly bend at the waist, bending your right knee as much as you need to allow you to touch your forehead to your right knee. The objective is not to overstretch the lower back but rather to feel a stretch in your extended leg. To deepen the pose, flex the right foot so that the toes curl toward you, straighten the leg, tuck the elbows in toward the body, and pull the elbows down toward the floor. Use your breath to deepen the pose by inhaling as you hold the stretch, and exhaling as you go deeper into the stretch. Be very careful to move slowly in this pose, allowing for the discomfort of the stretch without forcing the lower back to overstretch.

After holding the pose for at least five slow counts, slowly roll up the spine and repeat for the left leg. Stay on the floor and transition into Cobra Pose.

8. Cobra Pose

Lie belly down on the floor with hands at your sides and legs completely extended, feet together and tops of your toes resting on the floor. Resting your chin on the floor, bend your arms so that your hands rest close to your chest, fingertips facing forward. Tighten the buttocks, press the feet into the floor and slowly lift your head so that your gaze begins to travel first outward, then upward toward the ceiling. As your head begins to move up, begin pushing with your forearms (while keeping your pelvis pressed towards the floor) and allow the chest to lift off of the floor like a cobra. Be very careful to move slowly and deliberately. If you feel a pinch in your lower back, lower the chest back towards the floor and make sure you are keeping your seat firmly contracted. Try to keep your forehead relaxed (rather than furrowing your brow) and remember to gently rest the back of your head onto your neck. In its fully extended position, your forearm and upper arm should form no greater than a ninety-degree angle. Hold this position for at least five counts, using the breath to sustain you in the pose. Then slowly lower the chest until it rests onto the floor, and transition into the final resting pose, Corpse Pose.

9. Corpse Pose

Some say this pose is the most difficult for Westerners, because it asks us to be completely still (which really challenges our modern impatience!). Lie on your back, arms at your sides and palms facing upward, legs fully extended and heels lightly touching. Take five full belly breaths, allowing the abdomen to rise and fall with each breath. As each breath is released, see if you can let go of tension and allow the floor to support your weight. Stay in this position as long as you need to fully reap the benefits of the exertion and rest of your Yoga postures, then roll on your side and slowly come to an upright (seated) position before you get back on your feet.

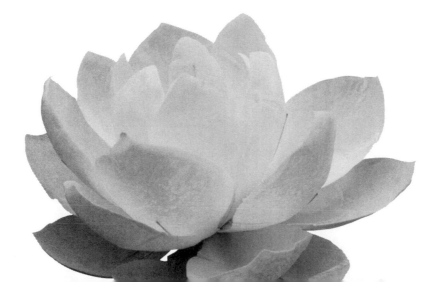

PART FIVE

Using the Cornerstones
of Balance

. . . When stillness comes
and my layers hold connected
I know peace.

17

ॐ

A Rhythm of Self-Care

In his book *Ayurveda: A Way of Life,* Dr. Vinod Verma emphasizes an Ayurvedic practice focusing on medicinal needs, cleansing, and revitalization. He writes that in Ayurveda, unlike Western medicine, the mind and body are not separated when considering treatment of an imbalance. All aspects of treatment—spiritual, rational, and psychological—are interdisciplinary, and as one area is affected, so eventually all areas are affected; in other words, restless minds affect health and happiness.[19]

However, when Westerners examine classic Ayurvedic treatments, the more esoteric aspects affecting spiritual health are sometimes difficult to relate to: gemstones, mantras, and the performance of atonements and cleansing rituals are not as easily acceptable to our rational minds. On the other hand, the use of diet and herbs, or the prescribing of certain Yoga postures to affect physical health, are more easily understood and assimilated. And yet the spiritual and psychological aspects, if examined from a more general point of view, are also readily applied to daily modern life.

Verma reminds us that the overuse of the mind and senses (such as watching violent movies, excessive worrying, and nonstop thinking) can lead to imbalance, and certain practices such as massage, meditation, Yoga postures, and breathing exercises help to revitalize both mind and body. What we see and sense evokes emotion and, therefore, creates subtle but accumulative physiological changes in the body.

Maya Tiwari, in *Ayurveda, a Life of Balance*, suggests that a key aspect of the spiritual nature of an Ayurvedic practice is a positive, grateful state of mind consciously created while doing daily activities.[20] Tiwari urges us to develop a sense of grace and gratefulness in receiving sustenance. Preparing meals, cleaning up, savoring food, sharing food, and growing food are all ways in which we may demonstrate thankfulness for the abundance we enjoy. Approaching food with the attitude of love and kindness, focusing on simple kitchens with simple tools and reducing toxicity in food by cooking with organic ingredients, less technology, and more thankfulness are all ways we may allow abundance into our lives.

Sally Morningstar, in *The New Life Library: Ayurveda,* describes how the use of aromas, massage, massage oils, colors, and herbal teas feed our senses with restorative, pleasing sensations.[21] Morningstar offers specific suggestions for nurturing and revitalizing each mind-body type.

For Vata

- Incorporate consistency into daily habits

- Eat warming food served in regular, sit-down meals

- Engage in gentle exercise to calm the mind without overdoing physical exertion

- Consume limited quantities of meat, poultry, and fish (if necessary) to help feel grounded

- Use daily self-massage of feet, hands, and head every morning, and a full-body massage weekly (massage benefits all mind-body types, but Morningstar suggests that the quality of Vata is particularly most benefitted by massage)

- Create environments with warming and gentle colors such as pastels or ochre, brown, and yellow.

For Pitta

■ Focus on gaining tolerance rather than feeling irritated and abrupt

■ Avoid spicy, fried, sour, or hot foods

■ Engage in vigorous and challenging exercise or sport,
but play games for enjoyment, not to win

■ Enjoy shaded and naturally calming surroundings, and use blues,
greens, and violets to appeal to the Pitta need for cool and calm

For Kapha

■ Learn to trust rather than holding on to stubborness, possessiveness,
and jealousy

■ Choose light, dry, hot, and stimulating foods

■ Build up self-discipline for vigorous, regular exercise

■ Use bright, invigorating colors such as red, orange, and pink
to stimulate the senses

■ Avoid overuse of the senses that numb mind and body
(such as too much television or overeating)

Morningstar also suggests that excess cold water, tea, coffee, and alcohol puts strain on the kidneys, as well as salt, sugar, and excess dairy and foods rich in calcium such as spinach. In other words, too much of a good thing is not a good thing. In her book, Morningstar discusses how to balance constitutions that have dual doshas or mind-body types, focusing on gaining a sense of seasonal awareness to appease the particular constitutional aspect. For example, a person with a Vata/Pitta constitution should avoid excessive heat in summer and extreme cold in winter—a suggestion that appeals to common sense as much as it does to an Ayurvedic practice.

Most of the suggestions for daily habits or "practices" are not created by Ayurveda but rather are inherent in our particular constitution's natural inclinations when in balance. Any gardener can tell you how growing vegetables or flowers heightens the appreciation for beauty and sustenance. Anyone with a Pitta constitution may reach an awareness that it feels better to be in sync with other people and the environment than constantly irritated, impatient, and ill-tempered. And if given a chance, we may all feel the effects of the seasons in a more comfortable way, rather than struggling to control our environments and our health.

Dr. Deepak Chopra suggests in *Perfect Health: The Complete Mind-Body Guide,* that we do not simply exist in our bodies, but in the natural environment around us.[22] We sense rain in our bones, we get restless with spring, we get lazy in warm weather, and our bodies change with the changes around us. Weather affects our constitutions, too: Vata increases with cold, dry, or windy weather; Pitta increases with hot, especially humid weather; Kapha increases with winter's rain and snow. Therefore in the spring and early summer, when Kapha influences are prevalent, we naturally prefer lighter, drier foods, less dairy, and warm food and drink with bitter, pungent, and astringent tastes. Midsummer through early autumn is a time when appetite naturally decreases due to hot weather, and cool food and drink is preferred (but not cold drinks as they diminish digestive fire). And in the Vata season, which goes from late autumn through winter, heavier and warmer food and drink are preferred, including use of more oils and the tastes of sweet, sour, and salty. Appetites may increase during this time of the year, which is why a regular exercise routine and balanced nutrition are important in helping us to not take in more calories than we can comfortably consume. With today's climate-controlled indoor environments, the appetite is more regulated since we are not subjected to as many extremes in temperature and weather.

Seasonality also goes into the realm of the practical: completing major yard projects in the hot, summer sun greatly increases Pitta, as well as vigorous hiking or biking midday, when the sun is at its peak. Working past the point of dinner into the late evening or night also puts Pitta on overdrive, and not making time for regular meals and self-nurturing keeps Vata jumpy. Pushing Vata or Pitta too hard is usually an invitation for Kapha to rise up in overabundance, like a wet, heavy blanket putting out the fire or bearing down on nervous exhaustion. It all comes down to choice, deciding which elements you need day-to-day to create a sense of well-being and nurturing. Vatas love warm baths, Pittas benefit from cool and peaceful sunsets, and Kaphas enjoy making time for good friends and fellowship. Finding what nurtures and appeals is the invitation of Ayurveda; Vatas may view it as a desirable way to increase comfort, Pittas may enjoy the challenge and resulting rewards, and Kaphas may look forward to increasing the variety of truly satisfying choices. Whatever approach best appeals to you, a look at your particular rhythm (or perhaps arrhythmia) may reveal opportunities to create a smoother, more balanced approach to your daily routine, and even to major life changes (which we often struggle with, rather than trying to understand). Finding the time to acquire new knowledge and habits, learning where to gain knowledge, and dealing with the impatience of our modern ways are challenges and obstacles to well-being, but also doorways to deeper self-understanding and skill.

Take a few moments and review the signs of imbalance you jotted down about your life at the end of chapter 4. These imbalances are doorways for growth, and the next and final chapter gives you an opportunity to use these observations about your life as starting points for the creation and strengthening of your cornerstones of personal balance.

18

𝒜

Your Personal Definition of Balance

Hunger is good when you hunger for that which nurtures you. Developing a rhythm of self-care means learning to satisfy your hungers by learning to create a sense of satisfaction that keeps your constitution in balance. Sometimes finding out what you need to stay in balance means becoming hungry for more knowledge and new ways of doing things—sometimes it means purposefully putting yourself out of balance until you know more about yourself and what you need. Seeking balance is not so much a matter of "laying low" and avoiding growth and challenge; rather, it's about developing stronger skills to help cope with the ups and downs of life, and gradually becoming more conscious of your needs so that you are able to make lifestyle choices which decrease the tendency for imbalance. Sometimes seeking balance means making hard decisions and undergoing big life changes, as well as paying attention to daily choices and unconscious habits.

As I began the transition from unconscious choice to having more clarity and skills to nurture myself in a more constructive and lasting way, my personal growth process took me into the realm of self-help. At first, my searching was more a process of learning who I wasn't, and, after countless lectures and seminars, workshops and retreats, healing circles and support groups, counseling and books, and lots and lots of introspection, I came to a point where I felt I had "unraveled" enough. First out of sheer need and then more and more out of an increasing sense of desire to be strong and well and more aware, I had opened myself up to new choices, and I began to develop the ability to listen to what my intellect, my heart, and my gut were trying to tell me about my life. As I listened more to my emerging inner voice, I began to benefit from the input of family, friends, and various teachers. Studying Ayurveda and engaging in a Yoga practice helped me to define the cornerstones I needed—and wanted—to create a more "well-fed" life; with this framework I was able to organize my thoughts more clearly and start making sense of all the growth and questions that had come from my process of personal struggle and inquiry. It was a bit scary to trust that I knew enough to begin making fundamental changes in my life, but it was also a relief. The self-help process can sometimes feel like a runaway train, moving too fast and taking too much of you with it. In fact, I've met some people whose passion is self-help, always in a state of inquiry but never developing their own sense of balance, relying instead on another's definition. In my case, I knew it was time to start pulling it all together when my desire for balance became a focal point in my actions and thoughts.

Consciously creating a sense of balance and well-being is a continuous process. Some of the "Eastern" approaches to wellness may be difficult to absorb, but we may find "teachers" everywhere, even in the unlikeliest of places. One of the best Yoga instructors I ever met could perhaps fit the stereotype of "way-out-there-hippie," with multiple body rings, ponytail, beard, purple tights, and, yes, even a tattoo—but he was very knowledgeable, articulate, compassionate, and extremely aware of each student in the class. Had I not allowed myself an open mind to learn about Yoga, I might not have realized the gifts that this particular instructor gave his students. An open mind allows you to gain greater awareness and new choices, but the point of Balancing is to develop a discerning mind so that you may make decisions based on an internal sense of values, not just someone else's viewpoint.

The process of Ayurvedic Balancing asks you to:

1. *Define what balance means to you by getting to know your particular mind-body constitution,* on physical as well as mental and emotional levels.

2. *Identify "hungers"* that are causing imbalance.

3. *Calm those hungers* through the cornerstones of balancing: Ayurvedic nutrition, exercise, relaxation and other self-nurturing practices, and actively engaging the imagination and intellect for healthy goal achievement.

Your Definition of Balance

Each part of this book has asked you to answer various questions concerning the concept of balance. Now it's time to identify goals and action steps to help you create a rhythm of self-care and build your own cornerstones of personal balance, based on your particular mind-body constitution. What action steps will you need to take to overcome obstacles and reach your goals?

Begin by listing three goals for each section, adding other goals as you either achieve the first goals, or as your priorities shift (see the chart on the following pages). Focusing on a few goals at a time greatly increases your ability to stay focused and achieve your objectives. Whenever possible, try to break a larger goal into smaller, more achievable steps. Take a few moments each week to review your progress, noticing if your personal belief system is helping or hindering the attainment of your goals, possibly inviting you to grow in another direction.

NUTRITION

What are my nutrition goals? Do they include a weight-management plan?
Are there other "hungers" I am feeling on a deeper level that affect my diet
and eating habits?

Goal	Obstacles	Actions
1. _____		
2. _____		
3. _____		

EXERCISE

What is my weekly exercise plan? Do I have any long-range goals for physical fitness, or current challenges that affect my fitness level? What skills do
I need to develop to reach my goals?

Goal	Obstacles	Actions
1. _____		
2. _____		
3. _____		

RELAXATION AND SELF-NURTURING

How may I specifically bring rest and relaxation into my daily life? How may I reduce the tension I feel in my life and increase my sense of inner well-being and peace?

Goal	Obstacles	Actions
1. ___		
2. ___		
3. ___		

Your Personal
Definition
of Balance

Continuing the Process

The more I continue to explore the concept of Ayurvedic Balancing from a personal perspective, the more I realize that Ayurvedic principles, which once seemed too esoteric and inaccessible, now seem a natural occurrence in day-to-day life. As we discussed in chapter 2, our state of being can be a marriage between what our bodies need and what our minds ask us to do. As we practice going in and out of Yoga poses, for example, we gain a larger analogy for moving through life: by learning to relax and restore ourselves after intense physical, mental, or emotional expenditures of energy, we help to keep ourselves in balance. Perhaps we can also learn how to not take our need for accomplishment and security so seriously that we get stuck in the "pose" of worry and tension and performance, missing out on enjoying the play and relaxation that we work so hard to earn.

Recently my neighbor and I were discussing my vegetable garden, and I told him that even though it sounds silly, I always get excited about having a lot of different vegetables ripen at the same time because it lets me eat abundantly as well as invite friends over for dinner or give them fresh produce. My neighbor, who is a professional chef by trade, commented that he understands more fully the Ayurvedic concept of creating abundance, simply by watching my enthusiasm for harvesting and sharing my garden's bounty. As he so eloquently summarized: "Cooking is more than the art of preparing a meal, it's a deepened appreciation for the growing, harvesting, savoring, and consumption of living food, and the love and affection which turns eating into nourishment." Coming from someone who is trained to prepare meat, heavy sauces, and gourmet desserts, I was touched that my simple yet undisguised enthusiasm for growing and preparing food had given him a sense of satisfaction and well-being. In other words, it doesn't take much for the simple pleasures of one's own life to positively affect another's. In creating abundance through my garden, the act of giving and sharing had become effortless, and self-fulfilling.

Creating abundance in life is like growing a very personal garden: you get to nurture your thoughts, emotions, and physical body, weeding out what doesn't work while observing which actions help you to grow and thrive. It's not an all-or-nothing process but rather an accumulation of knowledge and gradual changes over time. It's your garden—what would you like to grow?

References

Chapter 1

1. Tiwari, Maya. *Ayurveda: A Life of Balance.* Rochester, Vt.: Healing Arts Press, 1995, pp. 39–42.

Chapter 3

2. Svoboda, Dr. Robert E. *Prakriti, Revised Enlarged Second Edition.* Lotus Press, Twin Lakes, Wisc., 1998, p. 24.

Chapter 4

3. Morrison, Judith. *The Book of Ayurveda: a Holistic Approach to Health and Longevity.* New York, N.Y.: Simon & Schuster, 1995, pp. 64–65.

Chapter 5

4. Chopra, Deepak. *Perfect Health: the Complete Mind/Body Guide.* New York, N.Y.: Harmony Books, 1991, pp. 261–67.

Chapter 6

5. Kirschmann, Gayla J. and John D. *Nutrition Almanac*. New York, N.Y.: McGraw-Hill, 1996. Chapter 1 describes the process of metabolism and chapter 2 discusses target heart rate for fat-burning.

6. Ross, Julia. *The Diet Curse*. New York, N.Y.: Penguin Putnam, Inc., 1999. In particular, see chapter 2 on low-cal dieting and malnutrition and chapter 10 on nutritional rehabilitation for former dieters.

Chapter 7

7. Minirth, Frank, et al. *Love Hunger: Recovery from Food Addiction*. New York, N.Y.: Fawcett Columbine, 1990, p. 60.

Chapter 8

8. Moore, Thomas. *Care of the Soul: A Guide for Cultivating Depth and Sacredness in Everyday Life*. New York, N.Y.: Harper Collins, 1992, pp. 14–18.

9. Welwood, John. *Journey of the Heart*. New York, N.Y.: Harper Perennial, 1990, p. 5.

Chapter 9

10. Morningstar, Amadea. *Ayurvedic Cooking for Westerners*. Twin Lakes, Wisc.: Lotus Press, 1995, pp. 287–301.

Chapter 10

11. Rockwell, Sally. *The Coping with Candida Cookbook*. P.O. Box 31065, Seattle, Wash., 98103 (phone: 206-547-1814), pp. 2–6.

12. Morningstar, Amadea. *Ayurvedic Cooking for Westerners*. Twin Lakes, Wisc.: Lotus Press, 1995, pp. 232–35.

13. Chopra, Deepak. *Perfect Health: The Complete Mind/Body Guide.* New York, N.Y.: Harmony Books, 1991, pp. 256–57.

Chapter 11

14. Frawley, David. *Yoga and Ayurveda: Self-Healing and Self-Realization.* Twin Lakes, Wisc.: Lotus Press, 1999, p. 168.

Chapter 15

15. Richard Miller, Ph.D., personal correspondence, Nov. 1998.

Chapter 16

16. Chopra, Deepak. *Perfect Health: The Complete Mind/Body Guide.* New York, N.Y.: Harmony Books, 1991, pp. 42–45.

17. Richard Miller, Ph.D., personal correspondence, Nov. 1998.

Chapter 17

18. Verma, Vinod. *Ayurveda: A Way of Life.* York Beach, Maine: Samuel Weiser, Inc., 1995, Preface.

19. Tiwari, Maya. *Ayurveda: A Life of Balance.* Rochester, Vt.: Healing Arts Press, 1995, pp. 151–53.

20. Morningstar, Sally. *New Life Library: Ayurveda.* London, England: Lorenz Books, 1999, pp. 28–49.

21. Chopra, Deepak. *Perfect Health: The Complete Mind/Body Guide.* New York, N.Y.: Harmony Books, 1991, pp. 303–7.

Bibliography and Resources

Yoga Journal's *Yoga Basics* by Mara Carrico, et. al., New York, N.Y.: Henry Holt and Company, 1997.

> Good general descriptions of styles of Yoga, plus photos and instructions for various poses.

Perfect Health: The Complete Mind/Body Guide by Deepak Chopra, M.D., New York, N.Y.: Harmony Books, 1991.

> An easy to read, general introduction to Ayurveda with sections on diet and Yoga.

Yoga and Ayurveda: Self-Healing and Self-Realization by David Frawley, Twin Lakes, Wisc.: Lotus Press, 1999.

> This detailed book describes the relationship between Yoga and Ayurveda.

Nutrition Almanac by Gayla J. and John D. Kirschmann, New York, N.Y.: McGraw-Hill, 1996.

> Large, informative book that includes basic information on exercise and metabolism.

Richard Miller, Ph.D. Clinical psychologist, Yoga and meditation teacher, author and lecturer. (707) 824-1636.

Richard Miller was the co-founder of the International Association of Yoga Therapists, and is founding editor of the *Journal of IAYT.* He teaches throughout the United States and Canada.

Love Hunger: Recovery from Food Addiction by Dr. Frank Minirth, et. al., New York, N.Y.: Fawcett Columbine, 1990.

A comprehensive, step-by-step approach to identifying, understanding and healing addictive emotional connections to food.

Care of the Soul: A Guide for Cultivating Depth and Sacredness in Everyday Life by Thomas Moore, New York, N.Y.: HarperCollins, 1992.

A wonderfully written narrative about deeper, more soulful journeys in personal growth.

Ayurvedic Cooking for Westerners by Amadea Morningstar, Twin Lakes, Wisc.: Lotus Press, 1995.

Accessible introduction to Ayurvedic cooking, this book has a brief summary of Ayurvedic principles plus good recipes and interesting tidbits and comments from the author.

New Life Library: Ayurveda by Sally Morningstar, London: Anness Publishing, Ltd., 1999.

This colorful book details the Ayurvedic use of aromas, massage oils, colors, and herbal teas.

The Book of Ayurveda: a Holistic Approach to Health and Longevity by Judith H. Morrison, New York, N.Y.: Simon & Schuster, 1995.

This basic Ayurvedic text has lots of visual appeal.

The Coping with Candida Cookbook by Dr. Sally Rockwell, P.O. Box 31065, Seattle, Wash., 98103, 1996.

A short book about getting rid of yeast overgrowth using low-carb recipes.

The Diet Cure by Julia Ross, New York, N.Y.: Penguin Putnam, Inc., 1999.

An interesting dialogue about the disruptive effects of "dieting" on body chemistry.

Prakruti: Your Ayurvedic Constitution by Dr. Robert Svoboda, Albuquerque, New Mex.: Geocom, Ltd., 1991.

A short, concise, and insightful explanation of Ayurvedic terms and principles.

Ayurveda: A Life of Balance by Maya Tiwari, Rochester, Vt.: Healing Arts Press, 1995.

A large book containing in-depth psycho-spiritual descriptions of each mind-body type, plus recipes and personal, somewhat esoteric Ayurvedic practices for self-nurturing.

Ayurveda: A Way of Life by Dr. Vinod Verma, York Beach, Maine: Samuel Weiser, Inc., 1995.

This book is a detailed approach, discussing Ayurveda's background from Sanskrit texts.

Journey of the Heart by John Welwood, Ph.D., New York, N.Y.: Harper Perennial, 1990.

The subtitle to this book is "Intimate Relationship and the Path of Love." This book is an honest, well-presented discourse on the art of regaining intimacy in everyday life.

Index